D0555005

ACCLAIM FOR
The Healthcare Handbook

"At last, a book that helps patients navigate the healthcare system, assure that they get the most out of relationships with their healthcare providers, and have the tools to manage and direct their own health care outcomes. In her book, *The Healthcare Handbook: How to Avoid Medical Errors, Find the Best Doctors, Be Your Own Patient Advocate & Get the Most from Healthcare* Dr. van Servellen provides readers with the knowledge to not only increase their access to healthcare, but actively engage with and be heard by their providers to achieve quality care. The book delivers a toolkit for communication that offers practical approaches to establishing a collaborative relationship that makes the patient an active member of the healthcare team. It has long been the advice that patients and their families should be invested in the decisions about the what, when, and how of their healthcare – finally, Dr. van Servellen provides a way to make this happen. While this book is clearly needed by public consumers, it is also an excellent resource for the preparation of our health care professionals."

Judith F. Karshmer, PMHCNS-BC
Dean & Professor
School of Nursing & Health Professions,
University of San Francisco

"Dr. van Servellen presents an extremely valuable, timely, and easily readable guide for patients on the crucial process of achieving and maintaining quality health care. Her narrative is chock full of useful cutting edge information and resources. Starting with a brief review of current health care reform issues in the U.S., she provides important guides for recognizing quality care, understanding the roles of key primary care providers, selecting a good primary health care provider, nurturing an effective relationship, and communicating effectively. This highly useful guide to a challenging and evolving area belongs on the bookshelf of everyone concerned with maximizing the quality of their health care."

Theodore J Hahn, MD
Professor of Medicine, David Geffen School of Medicine,
University of California, Los Angeles

"Dr. van Servellen provides an excellent critical review of how various factors, such as the current healthcare system, clinician traits, and patient engagement and communication contribute to individual health care experiences. Useful tools and tips are identified so that readers can get the most out of their healthcare in the current changing environment. This book is timely and will be beneficial for readers looking to optimize the way they receive and obtain their care, as well as how they navigate the current health care system."

Jenice Guzman, PhD, RN
Gerontological Nurse Practitioner
Assistant Clinical Professor, UCLA School of Nursing

The Healthcare Handbook

How to Avoid Medical Errors, Find the Best Doctors, Be Your Own Patient Advocate & Get the Most from Healthcare

Gwen van Servellen RN, PhD

The Healthcare Handbook

How to Avoid Medical Errors, Find the Best Doctors, Be Your Own Patient Advocate & Get the Most from Healthcare

Gwen van Servellen, R.N., Ph.D.

Published by:

www.HealthcareBooks.net

ISBN: 978-0692262757

Copyright 2014 by Gwen van Servellen. All rights reserved. Unless otherwise noted, no part of this book may be reproduced, stored in a retrieval system, transmitted in any form or by any means, electronic, mechanical photocopying, or recording without express written permission from the author, except for brief quotations or critical reviews.

Disclaimer: The information and ideas in this book are for educational purposes only. This book is not intended to be a substitute for consulting with an appropriate health care provider. Any changes or additions to your medical care should be discussed with your physician. The authors and publisher disclaim any liability arising directly or indirectly from this book.

Other Selected Books by the Author

- *COMMUNICATION SKILLS FOR THE HEALTH CARE PROFESSIONAL: CONCEPTS and techniques (1st Edition)*
  Aspen Publishers

- *COMMUNICATION SKILLS FOR THE HEALTH CARE PROFESSIONAL: CONCEPTS, PRACTICES, AND EVIDENCE (2nd Edition)*
  Jones & Barlett, Publishers

TABLE OF CONTENTS

PREFACE AND ACKNOWLEDGEMENTS   xi

INTRODUCTION   xv

PART I: HEALTH CARE REFORM, QUALITY CARE, AND GETTING THE MOST OUT OF THE HEALTH CARE SYSTEM   xix

CHAPTER 1 Why Is Getting Quality Health Care a Problem?   1

- Factual Information About Health and Health Care   4
- Brief History of Health Care Reform, the Promises and Potential Problems   7
- Discussion of the Difference Between Access and Access to Quality Health Care   12

CHAPTER 2 Quality Care: We Know the Building Blocks and How to Get There   19

- Definition and Description of Quality Care   22
- Quality Care Ingredients   23
- Patient-Centered Care   23
- Continuity of Patient Care   24
- Coordinated Care   27
- Comprehensive Care   29

CHAPTER 3 Getting Safe Care: How to Prevent Errors From Happening to You   35

- What Is Unsafe Patient Care: Range of Potential Errors   38
- How to Be Your Own Best "Watch-Dog" and Make Your Care Safe   41

PART II: CHO0SING PRIMARY HEALTH CARE PROVIDERS 45

CHAPTER 4 Who are The Primary Health Care
Providers 47

- Roles of Providers Delivering Primary Care 50
- Family Practice Physicians (FPPs) 50
- Choosing the Appropriate Provider for You 55
- What Happens When You Do Not Have a Real
  Choice of Provider 58

CHAPTER 5 Criteria for Selecting a Good
Primary Care Provider 65

- What Are Primary Health Care Providers
  Authorized to Do 69
- What Standards Are They Held to 70
- Who Are the Good Providers According to Patients 70
- Who Are Good Providers According to Experts 73
- How to Choose a Primary Health Care Provider 74

CHAPTER 6 When to Select a Different Provider 83

- When to Change Providers 86
- Description of Traits in a "Not So Good and Bad Provider" 87
- Patients Report Complaints: How to
  Process These Complaints 88
- Selecting Another Provider 90

CHAPTER 7 Health Care Providers Are Human Too: Nurture
These Relationships 93

- Health Providers Want a Collaborative Relationship 96
- Are You Annoying Or Making Your Provider
  Upset Or Angry? 98
- How Do You Repair Your Relationship
  with Your Provider 100

**PART III: SKILLS TO WORK COLLABORATIVELY
WITH YOUR PRIMARY CARE PROVIDER**   103

CHAPTER 8 Communicating Successfully with Your
      Health Care Providers   105

  • Collaboration with Your Providers Requires Effective
    Communication   108

  • Principles of Communication and Your Role in
    Effectively Communicating   109

  • Help Reduce Errors by Shaping and Reshaping
    Discussions with Providers   112

  • Useful Tools You Will Want to Use Over and Over   115

CHAPTER 9 Managing Your Health Care and Treatment
      Effectively   121

  • What Are Your Responsibilities in Managing
    Your Health Care   124

  • Managing the Assessment and Treatment of Your
    Health and Medical Conditions   126

  • Why *Treatment Adherence* Is So Important   130

CHAPTER 10 Keeping Your Health Care Records and
      Coordinating Your Care   137

  • Quality Care Is Dependent Upon Your Care
    Being Coordinated   140

  • Tools Available to Ensure Your Care Is Appropriately
    Coordinated   140

  • How You Can Protect the Privacy
    of Delicate Information   147

**PART IV: SUPPLEMENT YOUR KNOWLEDGE
OF YOUR RIGHTS AND HEALTH CARE NEEDS**   151

CHAPTER 11 Your Health Care Rights and Responsibilities   153

  • General Description of Patient Rights
    in Health Care   156

- The Privileged Nature of Patient-Provider Relationship   157
- Patient Rights to Confidentiality,
  Anonymity, and Privacy   159

CHAPTER 12 Using Information Resources and the Internet
Wisely to Know About Your Health
and Health Care   165

- Warning Signs About Using Web Sites   168
- A Description of the Variety
  of Information Available   170
- How to Evaluate the Quality
  of Web Information   172
- How to Interact with Your Provider About Information
  On the Web   174

ABOUT THE AUTHOR   181

PREFACE AND ACKNOWLEDGEMENTS

Being able to communicate effectively and fend off potential medical mishaps is a must. The purpose of this book is to (1) provide you with the tools you need to actively engage in your overall health care, (2) address your concerns in finding and receiving high quality care, and (3) educate you on both a basic and advanced level. With the implementation of health care reform and the concern to provide not only access to care, but access to *quality health care*, this is a useful tool.

In short, this book will help you effectively navigate the health care system and avoid mishaps that can occur. Like most people, your knowledge may be limited and you may have trouble making sense of the sea of confusion in managing the care of yourself and your loved ones.

This book will teach you:

1. The major health care problems we face and the goals of national health care reform

2. What quality care is about

3. Sources of medical errors, and your role in preventing them

4. How to find and choose the best primary health care providers

5. How to communicate effectively with your health providers

6. Scripts you can use with your provider to prevent diagnostic errors

7. How to manage your health care and treatment effectively

8. Tools to maintain accurate health care records

9. Your rights as a patient

10. How to use the internet to find accurate and reliable health care information

The information presented here is particularly useful to those who are looking for primary health care services to meet their own needs and to those who are responsible for helping family members who require comprehensive health care, are sick, or require recovery care due to pre-existing conditions.

It is easy to understand the "why me" of this book; I pursued a career in health care with the dedication "to help people." My former students, patients, and professional peers gave me inspiration to put it in writing hoping to link new found access to high quality care. The idea, in fact, came from an observant reader; to paraphrase "….you can educate providers… but what about patients (providing this same information)? You might get further in educating patients… to create real change".

Intention must be combined with a wide range of advanced knowledge. As an internationally and nationally recognized educator, consultant, and author, I have over 35 years of experience observing, delivering, and evaluating quality and safe patient care. The latest of my books prepares health professionals to communicate effectively with patients for the purpose of ensuring high quality safe patient care.

The input of patients, students, medical providers, and scholars was priceless in creating this in-depth guide to getting the quality of care we all deserve. I relied heavily on their wisdom and a search of the literature on quality and safety of patient care, denying no spoken or written word the attention it deserved.

Several peers, family members, and friends helped along the way. Special thanks to Marissa Jones, BA, MS whose editing skills saw changes to be made and language to substitute. Also, to Joanne Douthat, BA whose astute editing of the book, along with Marissa's, brought out the essence of what patients and their families should know. Aline Stickler, BS, Training Specialist gave invaluable advice and information about the implementation of the ACA.

Additional thanks to colleagues for their contributions in the areas of quality care, health care systems, primary care, and remote care management of those with complex chronic illnesses:

- Judith F. Karshmer, PhD, PMHCNS-BC, Professor and Dean School of Nursing and Health Professions, University of San Francisco

- Donna McNeese Smith, EdD, RN, Professor Emeritus, School of Nursing, UCLA and specialist in health care systems

- Theodore J. Hahn, MD, Professor of Medicine, David Geffen School of Medicine, University of California, Los Angeles

- Jenice Guzman-Clark, PhD, RN, Gerontological Nurse Practitioner and nurse researcher, Veteran's Administration Greater Los Angeles Area and Health Care Center, Geriatric Research Education and Clinical Centers

INTRODUCTION

"It's not only about access to health care;
it's about access to quality care."

The Author

As miraculous as our ability is to diagnose and deliver some of the best medical care ever, providing access to high quality care remains a major barrier. Center stage is the newly implemented health care reform act. This provision is being rolled out in stages with the first being widespread insurance coverage for all US citizens. By now, you have had your own first hand experience with how the system works. As would be expected, such large scale change has its growing pains; reforms such as Social Security, Medicare, and Franklin D. Roosevelt's the New Deal of 1933-1933 were complicated programs as well and needed continuous refinement.

While access to health care is of current and major concern it tends to draw our attention away from the quality of care provided. With this said, we need to remember that quality care is an underlying issue that has haunted us for ages. So the issue is not just access alone, but equitable access to the best care possible. To this end I dedicate my time and commitment.

Problems with access to quality care have dominated health care both nationally and internationally. Examples abound, with current attempts to improve access present in recent legislation calling for health care reform. Recognized economic constraints are most important, as is the preparation of patients and health care providers to effectively partner to accomplish accessible high quality care.

The purpose of this book is to double your chances to effectively navigate the health care system and secure your rights to quality primary health care. The book is more about getting the most from health care than just surviving the health care system. Quality primary care helps you to prevent illness and recover more quickly when you are sick. There are many tips and pointers to help you achieve quality care in each and every chapter of the book.

Patient-provider collaboration in primary care is critical. Without this collaboration the risk of poorly involved patients and ill-equipped providers will defeat our health reform programs. Thus, health care reform may improve access, but, if not implemented carefully, may not fully address your needs for quality care.

The contents of the book include a broad range of facts and tips. First, you will be introduced to a brief background of the health care system and goals of the national health care reform. You may feel fully informed on this content; however, the information included in Chapter 1 draws on more than what health care reform is. You will be alerted to both the promises and some of the potential limitations of this reform. Following this backdrop you will learn what it takes to achieve not just access, but access to quality care.

The book devotes a substantial amount of attention to explaining the several factors leading to quality care, preventing medical errors, and how patients can protect themselves from the common mishaps. Being active in your health care and involving your family and care givers is foundational. An extremely useful and pragmatic part of the book will address how to communicate effectively and build good relationships with your providers. The two worlds of providers and patients will highlight why problems sometimes arise in your relationships and what you can do to resolve them.

There are many take-home messages and useful how-to-do-it descriptions in this book. They include:

1. A description of the history of health care reform, the U.S. National Health Care Reform Act and its potential promises and limitations

2. Definitions and descriptions of quality care

3. Details about the range of errors leading to patient injury

4. Description of primary care providers and their credentials

5. Guides to selecting a "good" primary health care provider

6. Guides in deciding when to seek a different provider

7. Ways to nurture your relationships with your providers

8. How to communicate effectively with providers

9. Managing your health and medical care in the stages of assessment, planning and implementing, and evaluating outcomes

10. How to keep and manage your personal health care records

11. Your basic rights as a patient receiving health care, including confidentiality, privacy, informed consent, and informed choice

12. Guides to using internet sources and websites as a resource for health care information, standard treatments, and provider reviews

The training and education of health care providers is perhaps the best yet. Unfortunately, there is a notable deficiency in the public's ability to understand, follow, and navigate health care delivery. In fact, improving the public's health care knowledge is a major goal of the nation's

Healthy People 2010 and the Institute of Medicine (IOM) report. Alarmingly, knowledge and skill which enables you to navigate the health care system effectively are ***absent in more than half of the U.S. population***.[1] This finding is disturbing because having this knowledge and skill can lead to longer life, improved quality of life, reductions in troubling effects of chronic and acute illness, as well as cost savings. The intent of this book is to better prepare you for active participation in the health care you choose, purchase, and receive.

REFERENCES

1. Institute of Medicine of the National Academies. *Health Literacy A Prescription to End Confusion.* Washington, D.C.: The National Academies Press. Available at: *www.nap.edu.*

PART I

- Why is getting quality health care a problem

- Quality care: We know the building blocks and how to get there

- Getting safe care: How to prevent errors from happening to you

CHAPTER 1

WHY IS GETTING QUALITY HEALTH CARE A PROBLEM?

*In the past, the benefits of modern medical science have not
been enjoyed by our citizens with any degree of equality.
Nor are they today. Nor will they be in the future--unless
government is bold enough to do something about it. Every
American has a right to affordable, high-quality health care.*

President Harry S. Truman
In an address to Congress, November 19, 1945

WHAT YOU'LL FIND IN THIS CHAPTER:

- **FACTUAL INFORMATION ABOUT HEALTH AND HEALTH CARE**

- **BRIEF HISTORY OF HEALTH CARE REFORM, THE PROMISES AND POTENTIAL PROBLEMS**

- **DISCUSSION OF THE DIFFERENCE BETWEEN ACCESS AND ACCESS TO *QUALITY* HEALTH CARE**

We don't necessarily want to hear it:

- How unhealthy we are
- How many people are getting no or inadequate health care
- How no or poor access to care leads to early mortality rates
- What it's going to take to turn this situation around

There is a need for everyone to become better informed. A better understanding of health care needs and problems will better prepare you to get the most out of the health care system. The information in this chapter will summarize for you important data about the nation's health and health care, what health care reform means, and how the U.S. and other countries have positioned themselves to provide health care equity. Lastly, you will learn the philosophy behind collaborating with your health care providers to achieve quality care and how you can prepare for the challenges ahead for you and your family.

FACTUAL INFORMATION ABOUT HEALTH AND HEALTH CARE

Like all industrialized countries, the United States faces a significant threat from chronic diseases. Deaths from the rising prevalence of chronic diseases are alarming. The chronic diseases most likely to lead to mortality are heart disease, cancer, chronic obstructive pulmonary disease, and stroke.

However, these diseases can be prevented and early detection can reduce the number of deaths and negative impact on our quality of life. Here is some factual information worth knowing followed by a discussion of how health care reform, if successful, can reduce these threats. The following are some details about the major threats to our health and well-being: *

1. Heart disease, cancer, and chronic obstructive pulmonary disease are the three leading causes of death in the US.

4

2. One in every four deaths are due to heart disease and the most common type of heart disease (coronary heart disease) is estimated to cost the US $208.9 billion each year.

3. High blood pressure, high cholesterol (LDL), and smoking are key risk factors for heart disease and half of Americans have at least one of these risk factors, and many have two or three.

4. Cancer, the second leading cause of death, accounts for 23% of all deaths.

5. Cancer and heart disease together account for half of all deaths in the U.S. [1]

A closer look at the death rates across groups reveals that survival is unequally distributed across our population with deaths from major diseases varying by ethnicity and poverty level. Those impoverished and less advantaged are dying in greater numbers from these diseases than many of their more socially and economically privileged counterparts.

Preventive health care can and has improved the health of millions of people around the world and in the U. S. In many cases, access to health care has prevented major diseases and has significantly helped to treat disabilities and injuries. Technology to perform early diagnoses of illness and treatment has improved the quality of life and longevity of patients. Further, technology has also significantly contributed to the recovery and improved quality of life and longevity of persons already experiencing these serious illnesses.

Still, other developed countries have managed to achieve longer life expectancy, lower infant mortality, and better recovery rates from major diseases than the United States. Additionally, of the 33 developed countries, there has been only one without universal health care; this country was the United States. Those countries without some assurance of universal health care are primarily in parts of the Middle East and Africa where mortality is high and infectious diseases go unchecked.

Contrary to many assumptions, developed countries have implemented universal health care without resorting to "socialized medicine" per se. These programs are government supported, and in some cases privately funded, and maintain a commitment to provide medical care to everyone who needs it.[2]

Although health care reform happens everyday in the U.S., the commitment to provide health care to everyone who needs it has been appallingly absent. A united approach to address this commitment, as noted in the beginning of this chapter, has clearly lacked Congressional support as far back as the Truman administration 70 years ago.

According to the United States Census Bureau, 48.6 million people (15.7%) were without health insurance in 2011.[3] This figure did not change significantly in 2012 and varies across age groups and ethnicities. Factors impacting a decline in coverage include the recent economic crisis where not even routine care was something that many of us could afford. Significant numbers of people either delayed care when it was needed or went without any health care services.

Not only access, but the quality of care was also in question. Despite improved medical technology, the Institute of Medicine provided a two-part report (1999 and 2001) denouncing the alarmingly high rates of medical errors in hospitals.[4] In a separate study reported in 2013, medical errors was found to take 3rd place as a leading cause of death in hospitals.[5] These findings emphasize the need for patients to protect themselves and their families from harm and health care institutions to make patient safety a high priority. Prescription drug reactions and interactions, including fatal adverse drug reactions are difficult to estimate but believed to be a significant ongoing threat for patients in and outside the hospital.

*Note: These facts are compiled from data available through the Centers for Disease Control and Prevention (CDC), and various web sites for CDC. More information can be found through these sources and CDC's Center for Health Statistics.

Brief History Of Health Care Reform, The Promises And Potential Problems

Health care reform has a long history both in the U.S. and abroad. Every country with national health care coverage has undergone years of change in methods of delivering, organizing, and financing health care. "Universal" protection or coverage are now widespread in Europe and most or all people are covered. As for the U.S., in the same time period, the implementation of universal coverage has lagged behind.

Health Care Reform Milestones: There are many milestones dating back to the early nineteenth century that have impacted adoption of health care reform. For example, since the beginning of the nineteenth century and following WWII, President Harry S. Truman called for support of universal health insurance. Although there was recognition for the need of widespread health coverage before this, he was the first U.S. president to propose a plan for national health insurance. The proposal was defeated in Congress. Presidents since then, including both democratic (Kennedy, Johnson, and Carter) as well as republican presidents (Eisenhower and Nixon), viewed universal coverage as important. A major milestone in supporting national health care reform occurred in the Clinton administration in 1993-1994. This plan required every U.S. citizen and permanent resident to enroll in a health plan. It specified both minimum coverage and maximum out-of-pocket costs. People below a certain income were to pay nothing. Like other health reform proposals, the idea was to support national health care and control the costs to the average citizen or permanent resident. This bill was met with opposition from both republicans and democrats as alternatives were put forward. In 1994 the national health care bill was declared dead in the Senate.

Most recently the Patient Protection and Affordable Care Act (PPACA) (also referred to as the Affordable Care Act) has taken center stage. Previous attempts at reform had met with resistance and resulted in piece-meal changes to meet the needs of some but not all people. Private health insurance and Medicare, along with public sponsored health programs proved insufficient. Emergency room services had shown that they were inadequate in meeting patient needs, did not address the issue of preventive care, and costs were soaring astronomically. It was finally time to confront the need for major reform. Unlike previous attempts championed by presidential efforts, the ACA received congressional support and was signed into law March 23rd, 2010. Subsequent to its signing it was upheld as constitutional by the U.S. Supreme Court and has been on a path of scheduled implementation. President Obama is credited with the success of this proposal.

Goals for Reform: The ACA is constructed to address three major deficits in our current health care system. They are: *poor quality, inadequate access,* and *insurmountable health care costs.* These problems become more alarming when comparing the U.S. with other developed countries in which quality of and access to health care are better and costs are considerably lower. Under health care reform, quality goals will be addressed and will include a number of technological advances. These advances are likely to include: medical and health records all in one place; internet devices to analyze and track health changes; remote monitoring of your health and needs for medical visits; and monitoring quality of care through measures of the outcomes of this care. These technologies are described in the many chapters to follow.

Health Care Access is Foundational: Accessibility to affordable care is the foundation of current healthcare reform and is continuing to be rolled-out with the implementation of ACA. This statute requires every individual to carry health insurance. The number one change is that everyone (excluding undocumented immigrants) who wants health care insurance will be able to get it at, theoretically a better cost than what was previously the case. This means you are guaranteed the opportunity to enroll in a health plan. However, there are problems to be addressed. This care may be more costly in the short run. If you have had a plan in the past, new plans may be considerably better in coverage; however, the cost may also be higher. If you opt for a plan that is more comprehensive and meets newer requirements, the premium might be higher but the out-of-pocket costs less. A critical issue is the cancelation of coverage for some individuals whose previous plans did not meet ACA requirements. Some of these individuals were faced with the problem that new plans are more expensive than the cancelled plan. The Centers for Medicare and Medicaid Services (CMS) is in the process of making these individuals eligible for a hardship exemption; also, they will be able to enroll in catastrophic coverage only. In order to take advantage of this option, you would need to fill out a hardship exemption form and submit proof that your policy was cancelled.

How Insurance Costs Are Determined: The main difference between health insurance plans are in: premium costs, out-of-pocket expenses, and insurance deductible. Under the ACA, the *premium* (the monthly amount of money you and/or employer pays for your health care coverage) that you are charged is based upon what your insurer decides is adequate to cover your health care costs. Your insurance will come through your employer or through individual state officiated marketplaces according to mandated formulas. Your choices are limited to what plans are acceptable and these plans have fixed costs. When you go to a health care provider to receive services you may be charged a *co-payment*. A co-payment, or copay, is usually a minimum amount of the total charge for services due at time the service is given and is what is referred to as out-of-pocket expenses. Originally, copays were used to deter people from obtaining unnecessary services. With the passing of health care reform, copays have been regarded as barriers to many people who could not afford basic preventive health care. Hence, copays have been eliminated in some cases (e.g. for those obtaining preventive health care and annual checkups). Copays may not exist in some instances but still one needs to be aware of premium costs that could exceed the amount of $20 copays per visit annually for a family of four.

An additional insurance cost you should be aware of when choosing a plan is the health insurance *deductible*. An insurance deductible is an annual dollar amount that you must pay before your plan will contribute anything towards the costs of your care. With the exception of a large scale integrative health care system like the Veterans Health Administration (available only to veterans and their families) or Kaiser Permanente Senior Advantage HMO, most health care plans will have some level of deductible. Usually deductibles apply only to visits where some care is rendered for a specific condition. Standard office visits or routine checkups do not apply. When you receive care for a particular condition you are responsible for paying the first portion of treatment which may be over several visits. When you have reached the dollar amount of your deductible, the insurance company processes your bills to pay the remaining balance. The advantage to you of an annual deductible is that it may create a lower monthly health insurance premium making higher quality and more comprehensive policies more affordable for you.

The exact balance of premium costs, copays, deductibles and quality of insurance plan is complex. For this reason, your decisions are best made under the guidance of counseling of your representative. For example, if you get coverage from an Employer Sponsored plan your broker would be your resource for guidance or your human resources or HR department.

Financial Help for Insurance Costs: If you are applying for insurance through the state operated Health Insurance Marketplace, you will be able to enroll and tailor your options to meet your personal situation. Additionally, you should be able to find out, based upon your income and household basis, if you are eligible for financial assistance to cut your costs.

Under the Affordable Care Act you may or may not be eligible for financial relief. Americans making less than $45,960 (as an individual) or the equivalent of $94,200 (as a family of 4) may be eligible for free or low-cost health insurance due to cost assistance subsidies. These guidelines will fluctuate annually as it is determined by the Federal Poverty Level chart reviewed yearly by the Department of Health and Human Services. These premium costs and cost sharing subsidies lower cost sharing on copays, coinsurance, and deductibles. Those who are financially poor are obvious candidates. This relief would come in the terms of a federal subsidy or monetary assistance in buying your insurance and would be provided to you through tax credits. Otherwise, it is possible to receive deductions from your federal taxes (tax credit) to make it possible for you to afford insurance premiums.

Promises of ACA Are Significant: The promises of this new health care reform are significant. Not only will access to insurance be made easier for you, but you will no longer be discriminated against because of pre-existing conditions (e.g. a cancer, heart disease, stroke or other diseases of lesser severity, or projected diseases such as those genetically linked or familial conditions). Health insurance coverage will be available to you whether you have pre-existing conditions or are healthy. Additionally, children and young adults (up to 26 years of age) are able to stay on their parents' insurance plan. This change is particularly helpful to young adults having difficulty finding jobs in a financial recession. Also, none of your preventative care or annual checkups will be out-of-pocket expenses; otherwise, what we call "co-pays" will be significantly reduced or brought to zero.

ACA Not Without Problems: Although U.S. health care reform promises to bring about many improvements in health care, it is not without problems. First, not all people in the U.S. will have access to health care. Particularly, undocumented immigrants will not be eligible. How are they to have access to quality of care in a timely manner? Currently the answer lies in these individuals being allowed services through Emergency Room only or cash only clinics. While this solution is a viable one, it is uncertain that quality care will result from somewhat fragment encounters with health systems. Secondly, those who choose to decline health insurance will be subject to a tax. How will the careful collection of taxes be implemented and how will they get access to quality care?

Of significant concern and unknown are the projections of costs. Different organizations have come up with different projected costs, showing that there is no real agreement on how much the ACA will cost down the line. Still, the Congressional Budget Office is responsible for determining these figures and determined a cost figure prior to the ACA being passed. The CBO proposal was subsequently upheld by the Supreme Court.

DISCUSSION OF THE DIFFERENCE BETWEEN ACCESS AND ACCESS TO QUALITY HEALTH CARE

Since mandatory health insurance coverage is here, one of your tasks is to make an informed choice about the insurance policy for you. If you are faced with multiple options for coverage you will want to make sure that your choices provide you with the best quality care possible. One of the key features, and a requirement, of the ACA and small and large group health plan notices is that the information provided is presented in easy to understand plain language.

If you are seeking coverage through Health Insurance Exchanges these exchanges have the responsibility to answer questions and help you make informed decisions. Health Insurance Exchanges have the responsibility to answer questions you have related to the Exchange (or Marketplace). They cannot advise you on an Employer Sponsored plan. For this help it is important that you contact your HR department or broker.

If you are interested in seeking coverage through the Exchange or the Marketplace as an individual, you have several options. First, the Federal resource for information is found on the health care law and Marketplace website: *healthcare.gov*. Also, an individual can call, go online, or seek assistance via paper documents or, when available, through walk-in assistance centers.

Through *healthcare.gov* you can get help through the entire process from beginning to end with the information you provide over the phone. You will be able to review your options and actually receive help in enrolling in a plan. They can also answer your questions as you fill out the paperwork. You will be able to compare health insurance plans based not only on your health care wants, but also your health care needs. Help to complete the paperwork for enrollment in a plan is available to you 24/7 (the 24/7 hotline phone number is 1-800-318-2596; TTY: 1-855-889-4325). There are also representatives to "Chat online" via IM on the website. By calling or reaching out online, local in-person help can also be provided to individuals as well as to brokers, navigators, and assisters.

Also, you can compare plans on the basis of price, benefits covered, quality provided and other features. You can do this in the low-pressure environment of your home and even with friends and family that can help you sort through and make informed decisions about different companies and different options across plans within companies.

When you compare Marketplace insurance plans they are listed in 5 separate categories: *Bronze, Silver, Gold, Platinum, and Catastrophic.* When choosing your plan think about the health care needs of you and your household. For example, when you consider which Marketplace insurance plan to buy do you expect to have many doctor visits? Will you be needing regular prescriptions for medications? If you do then you may want a *Gold* or *Platinum* plan. If you don't, you may prefer a *Bronze* or *Silver* plan. But remember that if you do choose a *Bronze* or *Silver* plan and get into a serious accident or have an unexpected serious illness, these plans will require you to pay more of the costs.

The ACA compliant plans are mandated to cover the following health and medical care areas:

- Ambulatory care

- Emergency care

- Hospitalization

- Maternity and newborn

- Mental health and substance abuse care

- Prescription drugs

- Laboratory tests

- Prevention and wellness care

- Chronic illness management

- Rehabilitation and devices

- Pediatric care (including oral and vision care)

Overall, new regulations on insurance plans aimed at protecting consumers will be the most significant change in health care reform. As previously described, you will have access to insurance even with pre-existing health conditions without it costing more than if you had no pre-existing conditions. This change will significantly help those who previously were unable to receive care when they were so in need due to long term chronic illness or incomplete surgical recovery. Otherwise, important continuity of health care for these individuals will be made possible.

Access is important; however, access to quality health care is the prevailing concern. Knowledge and skill enabling you to navigate the health care system effectively and achieve quality care is absent in more than half of the U.S. population. This is most disturbing because having this knowledge and skill often leads to longer life, improved quality of life, reduction of the troubling effects of chronic and acute illness, as well as cost savings.

Getting the most out of health care today requires knowledge and skills in areas that may not be altogether familiar to you. You will be encouraged to assume an active role, to search information for answers, to collaborate with your providers, and ensure your care is coordinated. The current rapid pace of screening and caring for large numbers of patients necessitates that you accept the challenge.

The purpose of the following chapters is to provide you with information that will help you understand the health care system but also, so important, get quality care. While much of the content can apply to all areas of health care services, the focus is on primary care or outpatient care. Primary care is the *gatekeeper* to the health care system. When choosing a primary care provider you gain access to general health care, disease prevention, and monitoring of some chronic illnesses. Primary care is critical because it controls access to other health care institutions (e.g. hospitals, specialists, laboratory testing, and other medical services.

REFERENCES

1. Centers for Disease Control and Prevention. Data on chronic disease prevention and health promotion provided by the National Center for Health Statistics. Available at: http://www. cdc.gov/nchs. Accessed October 30, 2013. (Also see *FastStats.*)

2. Kaiser Health News. *Census: Number of People without Health Insurance in 2012.* Available at: www.kaiserhealthnews.org/Daily-Reports/2013/September/17/census-data-uninsured.aspx. Updated 9/17/13. Accessed October 30, 2013.

3. Reid TR. *The Healing of America: A Global Quest for Better, Cheaper, and Fairer Health Care.* New York, New York: Penquin Books; 2009, p. 3.

4. Institute of Medicine. *To Err is Human: Building a Safer Health System.* Released in November 1999 and *Crossing the Quality Chasm-A New Health System for the 21st Century.* Released March 2001. Available at: iomwww@nas. Accessed December 17, 2013.

5. James J. A new, evidence-based estimate of patient harms associated with hospital care. *J Qual Patient Saf*, 2013; 9(3)122-128.

RESOURCES

- Affordable Care Act: Full Text. Available at: http://docs.house. gov/energycommerce/ppacacon.pdf. Updated June 9, 2010. Accessed October 30, 2013. The Affordable Care Act (ACA) is contained in an immense 2,000 plus paged document too large to read and comprehend for most of us. But should you want to look at it and read sections this is the resource. There are several smaller condensed versions available online depending upon what your interest is.

- Kaiser Family Foundation Health Reform Source: http:// healthreform.kff.org/ and Kaiser Permanente. Find Out How Health Care Reform Affects You. Understanding the Affordable Care Act. http://healthreform.kff.org/.

- Medical News Today. Affordable Care Act Delivers Cheaper Prescription Drugs to Nearly 500,000 People. Available at: http://medicalnewstoday.com/releases/229881.php. Accessed September 4, 2013.

- Reid TR. *The Healing of America: A Global Quest for Better, Cheaper, and Fairer Health Care*. New York, New York: Penquin Books; 2009. This book is a New York Times Bestseller. It is an excellent resource for understanding the differences between our health care system compared to those in other countries. It illustrates how we can make use of the lessons learned from industrialized democracies whose health care is universal, affordable, and effective.

TERMS

Affordable Care Act (ACA): This is the term used to refer to recent health care reform legislation.

Co-Pays (Copayments): These payments represent a minimum amount of the costs of medical services given. They are due at the time of receiving medical care. Co-pays for preventive health care under health care reform in some instances will not be required.

Federal Subsidies: Federal subsidies refer to monetary relief to assist you in paying for health insurance.

Health Insurance Exchanges: Health reform legislation has created state-based health insurance exchanges. Individuals and small businesses can compare the costs of various health plans and different types of health coverage benefits. The purpose of the health insurance exchanges is to make health insurance more affordable and easier to purchase for small business and individuals.

Health Insurance Premium: This amount of money you and/or your employer pay (usually once a month) for your health care coverage.

Obamacare: The term used to refer to the Affordable Care Act.

Patient Protection and Affordable Care Act (PPACA): The full title of the ACA. PPACA, ACA, and Obamacare refer to the same legislation.

CHAPTER 2

QUALITY CARE: WE KNOW THE BUILDING BLOCKS AND HOW TO GET THERE

"Access to basic quality health care is one of the most important domestic issues facing our nation."

Edward Lopez Pastor
(Member of the U.S. House of Representatives
from Arizona since 1991)

Ed Pastor. (n.d.). BrainyQuote.com. Retrieved December 29, 2013, from BrainyQuote.com Web site: http://www.brainyquote.com/ quotes/quotes/e/edpastor377727.html

WHAT YOU'LL FIND IN THIS CHAPTER:

- **DEFINITION AND DESCRIPTION OF QUALITY CARE**

- **QUALITY CARE INGREDIENTS**

    - **PATIENT-CENTERED CARE**

    - **CONTINUITY OF PATIENT CARE**

    - **COORDINATED CARE**

    - **COMPREHENSIVE CARE**

It's no big secret. We know what quality patient care is. So why doesn't every patient receive quality care? The long and short of it is: resources... resources...resources...resources. Of course for some providers, hospitals, and insurance companies it is: profits...profits...profits. Regardless, of which or both, every patient is not receiving quality care.

Current health care reform is taking center-stage in promising better care. The primary goal of health care reform is to provide affordable health insurance for all U.S. citizens. Care that is accessible to all is the foundation for enhancing widespread quality care. However, access to care is insufficient. What about the quality of this care that is going to be made accessible? Getting quality health care helps you stay healthy and recover more quickly when you are sick. Obviously, we need to go beyond the issue of access and address key features of quality care.

The following is an in depth review of what quality care is and the specific features to look for. It will help you to know when you have it and when you don't.

DEFINITION AND DESCRIPTION OF QUALITY CARE

The Institute of Medicine (IOM), in its several reports on quality health care, defined quality as: "The degree to which health services for individuals and populations increase the likelihood of desired health outcomes and are consistent with current professional knowledge."[1] The IOM report defined quality care as being: safe, effective, patient-centered, timely, efficient, and equitable.

Quality care has long been the focus of health care planners and professionals. We know the characteristics of health care systems that promote quality. Quality health care is the result of superior levels of knowledge and skill in an environment of high intentions and sound decision-making. The characteristics that define a high-quality health care service include the following: patient-centered care, continuity care, coordinated care over time and across services, and comprehensive and accessible care. In the following discussion we will present these quality attributes, define them, and show you how you can identify these key components in the health care services you seek and receive.

QUALITY CARE INGREDIENTS

PATIENT-CENTERED CARE

The IOM (Institute of Medicine) defines patient-centered care as: *"Health care that establishes a partnership among practitioners, patients, and their families (when appropriate) to ensure that decisions respect patients' wants, needs, and preferences and that patients have the education and support they need to make decisions and participate in their own care".*[2]

Examples of patient-centered care in primary care include:

- Patient interviews that ask the patient to describe his/her health problem in detail
- Respect and appreciation of the patient's views in medical decision-making
- Recognition and respect for the patient's cultural traditions, personal preferences and values, lifestyle, family, and social circumstances
- Patient support and empowerment to participate actively in his/her care

What patient-centered care is not:

- The provider giving you whatever it is you ask for, including medications or procedures not medically warranted
- Over solicitous behaviors which take up necessary time and work against your ability to describe your problem and encourage the provider to really listen to you

- Abrupt responses that limit your story and your ability to explain how your symptoms have changed over time and affect your life
- Domination of the discussion of what it is you need without asking you your thoughts on how treatment should go

There are many examples of both good and bad patient-centered care. In the first few minutes of your appointment you may be able to judge just how patient-centered a provider is. You may have reactions that give you a hint about this very aspect about your care with the provider. Expected consequences of patient-centered care are:

- Better communication with your provider
- Higher provider effectiveness
- Improved incentives for the patient to participate effectively in care

Patient-centered care is linked with higher quality of care and higher patient satisfaction. It means treating the "whole person", not just the illness or injury bringing the patient to the office visit. While current health care reform measures are believed to increase patient-centered care, it is important that the consumer ensures that she/he receives care that is patient-centered.

CONTINUITY OF PATIENT CARE

According to the American Association of Family Physicians, *"Continuity of care is a hallmark and primary objective of family medicine and is consistent with quality patient care. The continuity of care inherent in family medicine helps family physicians gain their patients' confidence and enables family physicians to be more effective patient advocates."*[3,4] Research has linked continuity of care to patient satisfaction, decreased need for hospitalization and emergency room care, and improved delivery of preventative care. Continuity of care is cost-effective because it paves the way for early recognition of health care problems. Formerly rooted in a long-term relationship between patients and doctors, it ensures the integration of information over time.

Continuity of patient care can be relational or informational.

1. **Relational Continuity:** Care over time by a single individual or team of health care professionals with effective and timely communication of health information.

2. **Informational Continuity:** The careful transmission of medical information from one provider to the next.

Most patients know what continuity of care is not. Typically, continuity of care does not include having a serial list of providers to see within the same medical group and never knowing who you are likely to see next. A continuous relationship with a single provider is interrupted and may happen many times in the course of primary care visits. You need to understand what continuity means more generally and what you can expect.

There are very concrete examples of how continuity is manifested. The following are commonly observed in settings where there is very high continuity:

- Provider(s) know your name, your conditions, and the plan for your care.
- They also know the results of current treatments, what medications you are taking and what test results have shown.
- They are familiar with your specific culture, religious, and social details that influence your views and medical decisions.
- They see you frequently enough to have developed trust and good communication.
- Their conclusions during this visit incorporate many details found throughout the course of coming to see them.

On the contrary, concrete manifestations of poor continuity with a health care provider include:

- Frequent turnovers in those providers you see within the medical group.
- Difficulties in forming trusting relationships with the providers because you have never met them or have not seen them regularly (for example, the last time you saw them was a year ago).
- Communications remain superficial and brief because you lack the trust to confide in them.
- Instances in which providers make mistakes about your most current problem, your previous chronic illnesses, your current medications, or when you were last seen by them.

However, traditional forms of continuity of care (one doctor to one patient) are outdated. It has been replaced by a medical team and patient. Who will see the patient varies depending upon scheduling realities and needs of the patient. Continuity is preserved by medical records and plans of care maintained by the team who shares the same data, updates the information as needed, and who will see the patient.

Have we sacrificed continuity in our needs to give more care with increased numbers of patients and reduced numbers of providers? No, but we are likely to rely on informational continuity versus "old fashioned" relational continuity of care. Perhaps we can never go back to the time when the same provider sees the same patient over long periods of time but some providers try and, even out of necessity, they do (for example, in rural settings where there is a lack of providers for miles around). These providers are likely to tell you that they cherish the individual relationships they have with their patients and place a premium on relational continuity as an essential part of good patient care.

COORDINATED CARE

Coordinated care refers to linking health care services so as to reduce fragmented care. It is also known as integrated care or the delivery of seamless care. It is an increasing trend to devise organizational arrangements to achieve improvement of services. The World Health Organization defines integrated care as the following: *"Integrated care is a concept bringing together inputs, delivery, management and organization of services related to diagnosis, treatment, care, rehabilitation and health promotion."*[5]

To understand coordinated care you will need to also understand fragmented care. Fragmented simply means breaking off or rendering care in smaller parts. This can happen several ways in health care. For example, your care can be given by more than one or two providers. For a single condition you may be seeing your primary care provider and several specialists. When care is delivered by many providers including specialists, it may become fragmented with each provider paying attention to parts of your care but no one provider taking charge of the whole picture. Care can become fragmented within and across health care services (e.g. between two different providers within the same hospital or providers treating you for different illnesses). Fragmented care has been recognized as a major problem worldwide and is specifically addressed in recent health care reform.

Access to care through affordable insurance eliminates both not being able to be seen for treatment and having to shift in and out of different treatment facilities. Coordination provides necessary links between services across all aspects of care. For example, the idea is that specialty care (e.g. treatment by a cardiologist, hospital and home care treatment for cardiac problems, and medical support groups for heart valve replacement) would be effectively linked. All of these services would be coordinated by generalists (e.g. primary care providers) in a "medical home" system. These providers would talk to each other, medical records would be transferred across services aided by electronic medical records, and this entire effort would be housed in a virtual or real setting called a "medical home." The medical homes would be accountable for meeting the large majority of each patient's physical and mental health care needs; including prevention and wellness, acute care, and chronic illness care management. The medical home approach is particularly needed for patients with complex needs due to multiple chronic illnesses and health conditions.

The concept of health care providers and services working together in a coordinated fashion is critical to quality care. In the purest sense it is both horizontal (links similar levels of care, such as multi-professional teams) and vertical (links different levels of care, such as primary care with specialty and end-of-life care).

Examples of care that is coordinated include:

- Communication and collaboration between your primary care provider and your specialists (e.g. cardiologist)
- Electronic medical records linking your medical records with all other service providers caring for you (e.g. your medical, social, and psychological services)
- Communication and coordination between nursing care on two different hospital shifts

On the contrary, concrete manifestations of poor coordination of care would be:

- Failure to transfer medical records to and from different health care providers
- Miscommunications about important details about you and your care (e.g. current medications you are taking or your reactions to previous treatments)
- Problems in communication between a group of providers responsible for advising you about medical care options

One of the goals of health care reform is to coordinate care across all elements of the broader health care system, including: specialty care, hospitals, home health care, and community services and supports. Such coordination is particularly critical during transitions between sites of care, (such as when patients are being discharged from the hospital). Many medical errors are associated with poor coordination and have been linked to unnecessary re-hospitalizations or failure of treatment due to the fact that one set of providers is poorly informed about the opinions and directions of the other set of providers or treatment site. Also, the absence of coordination also is much more expensive. It is possible that some elders and the poor who seek emergency care frequently would go to different ERs making coordination of their care difficult.

One-stop shops or HMO provider practices offer a unique opportunity to ensure coordinated care. Kaiser Permanente Hospitals and Clinics, for example, provides care in all categories (preventive, chronic care management, and prescription services in one place). Their combined staff of doctors, specialists, nurses, laboratory staff, and pharmacists all work together under one roof. This is also true for VA health services.

COMPREHENSIVE CARE

Comprehensive care refers to the treatment of the whole patient, not just the disease, a part of the body, or a single episode of illness. It is sometimes referred to as holistic medicine because in this practice of medicine all aspects of the patient are considered relevant and are assessed and treated. This would include any concerns of a physical, psychological, social, and spiritual nature connected to the patient's condition.

Providing comprehensive care can require a team of care providers. This team might include physicians, advanced practice nurses (NPs), physician assistants, nurses, pharmacists, nutritionists, alternative medicine providers, social workers, educators, and care coordinators. Although some medical home practices may bring together large and diverse teams of care providers to meet the needs of their patients, many others, including smaller practices, will build virtual teams linking themselves and their patients to providers and services in their communities and beyond. Examples of services that are comprehensive care centered would include the following:

- Individual providers that address a wide range of patient needs (e.g. physical, psychological, social, and spiritual patient concerns).
- Teams of different specialists acting together to provide input and assistance with a complex health care condition (e.g. heart disease, cancer, and stroke).
- Linkages between community service agencies and medical services to provide the most up-to-date information about diseases impacting people in the local community.

Examples of services that are not comprehensive care centered include:

- Providers that treat only one aspect of your condition without concerning themselves with other aspects that might bother or worry you. For example, those that would treat a severe burn or injury from a physical and medical approach without addressing any psychological reactions you might have.
- Different specialists involved in your care unable to communicate among themselves because they do not value input from a broad range of views.
- Lack of public health programs to connect religious, medical, and community leaders with the needs of the community for health promotion and disease prevention.

Access to care is foundational to the delivery of quality care. Without it, quality can't be achieved. When care is in place, other principles of quality (e.g. patient-centered, continuous, coordinated, and comprehensive care), can take center-stage.

REFERENCES

1. Institute of Medicine. *Crossing the Quality Chasm: A New Health System of the 21st Century.* Committee on Quality of Health Care in America, Institute of Medicine. Washington, D.C.: National Academy Press. Available at: iom.www@nas. edu. Accessed October 18, 2013.

2. Institute of Medicine. *Crossing the Quality Chasm: A New Health System of the 21st Century.* Committee on Quality of Health Care in America, Institute of Medicine. Washington, D.C.: National Academy Press. Available at: iom.www@nas. edu. Accessed October 18, 2013.

3. American Association of Family Physicians. Continuity of Care, Definition of. Available at: aafp.org. Accessed November 1, 2013.

4. Sharma G, Fletcher KE. et al. Continuity of outpatient and inpatient care by primary care physicians for hospitalized older adults. *JAMA.* 2009; 301(16):1671-1680. doi:10.1001/ jama.2009.517.REE

5. Gröne O, Garcia-Barbero M. *Trends in Integrated Care – Reflections on Conceptual Issues.* World Health Organization, Copenhagen, 2002, EUR/02/5037864.

RESOURCES

- Agency for Healthcare Research and Quality. *Guide to Health Care Quality: How to know it when you see it.* Available at: www.ahrq.gov. Accessed November 17, 2013. This booklet outlines a number of pointers describing how you can take charge of your health care and ensure you get the highest quality you can find. Topics include finding quality information, understanding consumer ratings of care, and local regional and national organizations that support resources to promote your finding quality providers and medical services.

- American Academy of Family Physicians, American Academy of Pediatrics, American College of Physicians, & American Osteopathic Association. Joint principles of the patient-centered medical home. Available at: http://www.acponline.org/...demonstrations/jointprinc_05_17.pdf. Updated March 7, 2007. Accessed October 30, 2013.

- Center for Policy Studies in Family Medicine and Primary Care. The patient centered medical home: history, seven core features, evidence and transformational change. Washington DC: Robert Graham Center. Available at: www.graham-center.org. Updated November 2007. Accessed October 30, 3013.

TERMS

Comprehensive Care: Comprehensive care refers to the treatment of the whole patient, not just the disease, a part of the body, or a single episode of illness. It is sometimes referred to as holistic medicine because in this practice of medicine all aspects of the patient is considered relevant and is assessed and treated.

Continuity of Patient Care: The American Association of Family Physicians defines continuity of care in the following way: Continuity of care is a hallmark and primary objective of family medicine and is consistent with quality patient care. The continuity of care inherent in family medicine helps family physicians gain their patients' confidence and enables family physicians to be more effective patient advocates.

Coordinated Care: Coordinated care refers to linking health care services so as to reduce fragmented care. See Integrated Care.

Integrated Care: WHO describes integrated care as a concept bringing together inputs, delivery, management and organization of services related to diagnosis, treatment, care, rehabilitation and health promotion.

Patient-Centered Care: The Institute of Medicine describes patient-centered care as: Health care that establishes a partnership among practitioners, patients, and their families (when appropriate) to ensure that decisions respect patients' wants, needs, and preferences and that patients have the education and support they need to make decisions and participate in their own care.

Quality Care: The Institute of Medicine (IOM) in its several reports on quality health care defined quality as: The degree to which health services for individuals and populations increase the likelihood of desired health outcomes and are consistent with current professional knowledge.

CHAPTER 3

GETTING SAFE CARE: HOW TO PREVENT ERRORS FROM HAPPENING TO YOU

"You may not be injured or killed but even with the slightest chance you want to know what can go wrong in the health care system."

The Author

WHAT YOU'LL FIND IN THIS CHAPTER:

- **WHAT IS UNSAFE PATIENT CARE: RANGE OF POTENTIONAL ERRORS**

- **HOW TO BE YOUR OWN BEST "WATCH-DOG" AND MAKE YOUR CARE SAFE**

The Institute of Medicine's astonishing report about medical errors revealed an epidemic of errors that could be prevented.[1] The focus of this report was errors that occurred in hospitals. Errors in primary care or outpatient health care services were not addressed.

Now what appears to be the case is that errors occurring in outpatient settings (including primary care) are increasing and have accounted for more than half of the adverse events leading to malpractice claims in 2009. It is believed that these malpractice claims represent only the tip of the iceberg; the danger from medical errors in outpatient settings is far greater than what is known.

This chapter will help you avoid mishaps that can occur. Like most people your knowledge may be limited and you may have trouble navigating the sea of confusion in managing your care. This confusion can contribute to your fears that something may go wrong.

WHAT IS UNSAFE PATIENT CARE: RANGE OF POTENTIAL ERRORS

First of all, what is unsafe about patient care? Unsafe patient care is not just the absence of quality care. It is care that places you at risk for harm or even death. Unsafe patient care is more prevalent than you might know or even like to contemplate.

Errors that occur in hospitals have received the most attention and are possibly the most well known. You may have read or heard instances where doctors amputated the wrong leg in a surgical mishap, a patient eventually dying of bed sores and infections acquired in the hospital or nursing home, or a pediatric patient receives the wrong dose of a medication and dies.

There are numerous accounts that have gotten the attention of the news media. Recently, focus has been placed on the care that occurs in outpatient services. These services would be group or sole provider medical offices and outpatient *surgical suites*. An estimated 30 times more patient visits occur in outpatient services, so it could be that errors outside of the hospital may be even more serious than those that occur in hospitals. [2] Given these facts, it is important to arm yourself with the tools to identify the problem in your primary care provider arena. Medical errors in primary care can be grouped by category *and include diagnostic, medication, and treatment errors.*

Diagnostic errors (whether you are being evaluated appropriately) are high on the list in outpatient centers. The situation is complicated by the fact that an enormous number of tests are ordered and reports come back at varying times. If the provider is not on top of the data, important signs of disease and illness can be missed. With reduced time to spend with patients (and this may be reduced further with many more patients to see) even fairly obvious symptoms may be missed or patient stories be abbreviated, further jeopardizing quality assessments, diagnoses, and patient safety.

Medication errors have been and continue to be a significant problem. Primary care providers are known to rely heavily on the prescription of medications for treating patients with over half to two-thirds of patient visits resulting in the prescription or refill of at least one medication. Primary care providers spend a significant amount of time and effort in the refill of medications and many errors can occur. The types of errors providers expect to see are those in: prescribing (right medication and right dose to the right patient), filling and dispensing (pharmacy accurately fills the medication prescription), and monitoring effects and responding to reported symptoms (e.g. drug interactions that result from the patient taking the medication at the same time as other incompatible medications or over-the-counter formulas). Patient adherence to taking the prescribed medication is not a medication error but is extremely important. We address the issue of adherence to medications and treatments in Chapter 9.

Treatment errors have increased in numbers in primary care practices. Surgical outpatient services are receiving added attention. For some primary care offices, having surgical centers or rooms means an increase in revenue. Outpatient surgical centers, or even surgical rooms in provider offices, do not adhere to some of the quality control procedures found in hospitals. Further, they are not visited by state regulators who would ordinarily monitor for safe practices (such as in hospitals). This is a critical issue because many errors could be prevented with stronger oversight. This is one reason why the extent of medical errors in outpatient treatment, including private physician offices, is virtually unknown. The following discussion sharpens your awareness about what to look for and what medical errors mean.

Medical errors are an example of unsafe care. These errors can be either errors of omission (for example, a medication wasn't prescribed when it should have bee) or commission (something wasn't done right or should not have been done at all). Examples of errors of omission include some groups getting no treatment at all. One could say that health care reform measures are aiming to decrease these kinds of errors by providing more care to more people, particularly those who are vulnerable.

Errors of commission are actions taken that are not correct. Areas where this risk is high is in the prescription of medications or conducting certain treatments. Errors of this kind can cause injury, disability and even death. Prolonging illness or delaying recovery are consequences of mistreatment. Commission errors include mistakes in administering medications (e.g. to the wrong patient or the wrong dose to a patient requiring the medication). Though undesirable and unintentional, in either case, bad things happen or nearly happen.

Most medical errors can be prevented given what is known in medicine. Otherwise, they should not happen. Indeed, many providers already intercept great numbers of errors before they reach you and without you hearing about them. These may include errors in blood pressure readings and incorrect history taking including missing medications that have been discontinued.

How to be your own best "watch-dog"
and make your care safe

You are the consumer of outpatient primary health care services, whether they be in private or group medical offices, urgent care or surgical centers. It is imperative that you learn to differentiate between what are the good ones and what are the not so good ones.

Know that any of the categories of primary care providers listed in Chapter 5 have good and poor providers so looking at credentials alone will not ensure that you will avoid medical errors. How providers actually practice is critical. The most important skill and knowledge must support high quality diagnoses and management of health conditions. If they employ nonprofessional staff, these workers are not prepared to catch errors. If they do not practice according to research-based standards, their care is below par. Of course, they are human and all are subject to making mistakes. Be armed with knowledge. Here is a list of factors to consider when choosing your health care provider or health care provider group:

- What is their mission or purpose statement?
- Is safe care or quality care mentioned? Do they specify practicing according to safe and professional standards?
- How many nonprofessional staff are performing clinical care tasks?
- Does the provider perform procedures beyond his/her scope and level of training?
- Do you trust the manner in which your provider came to a decision about a diagnosis or need for therapy or treatment?
- How well are staff and providers explaining your condition, medical care and procedures?
- How well informed are your providers about alternative treatments and any consequences of the treatment they are prescribing for you?

- Are your requests for test results, health information, and referrals to specialists provided in a timely manner?
- Are medications described in full, including expected impact, potential side effects, and alternatives?
- Is the area in your receiving room kept clean and comfortable?
- Did your visit allow you the time to describe your concerns, tell the story of how you have felt, and ask questions?
- Were there any factors that prohibited your ability to talk openly and confidentially with your providers?
- If you brought a family member or friend along, were they given the opportunity to support you and, with your permission, a chance to ask questions of your provider?

Your providers should also be interested in your description of the most and least helpful aspects of your care and what can be done to improve your visits. If they are not, this does not mean they will deliver unsafe care, at least not initially. What it might mean is that because they have not bonded with you in a solid provider-patient relationship, they may miss critical data by virtue of not hearing your version of the symptoms you are experiencing.

In summary, while more of your care is being performed in outpatient settings, this does not mean your care is free of the typical errors reported about hospital care. In fact, it is more difficult to know what these errors might be and what is the probability that they might happen. Given these facts and the circumstances that quality and safety controls are not always followed or even in place, your role in protecting yourself is crucial. In some primary care practices, there are not the resources to address quality and safety issues. If simultaneously patients are seeing different providers who have not shared important information, it is possible that critical safety issues will fall through the cracks and put patients at further risk. Just exactly how successful we will be in reducing outpatient errors as we have reduced inpatient hospital errors is still unknown. A lot depends upon the quality of your communications with your providers and the extent to which your medical records are transmitted across your health care venues to eliminate poor coordination errors.

REFERENCES

1. Kohn LT, Corrigan JM, Donaldson MS. (Committee on Quality of Health Care in America) eds. *To Err Is Human: Building a Safer Health System*. Washington, D.C., Institute of Medicine, National Academy Press; 2000.

2. Wynia MK, Classen, DC. Improving ambulatory patient safety. Learning from the last decade, moving ahead in the next. *JAMA*. 2011;306(22):2504-2505. doi:10.1001/jama.2011.1820. Also see: American Medical Association. Research in Ambulatory Patient Safety 2000-2010: A 10-year Review. Available at: http//www.ama-assn.org. Accessed October 30, 2013. and Bishop TF, Ryan AM, Casalino LP. (2011). Paid malpractice claims for adverse events in inpatient and outpatient settings. *JAMA*. 2011; 305(23):2427-2431.

RESOURCES

• Agency for Health Care Quality and Research. Five Steps to Safer Health Care. Patient Fact Sheet. Available at: http//www.ahqr.org. Accessed October 30, 2013.

• Bishop TF, Ryan AM, Casalino L. Paid malpractice claims for adverse events in inpatient and outpatient settings. *JAMA*. 2011;305(23):2427-2431.

• Starfield B. Is US health really the best in the world? *JAMA*. 2000;284(4): 483-485.

TERMS

Diagnostic Errors: Diagnostic errors are those errors made in assessment and diagnosis of a health care or medical problem.

Errors of Commission: Errors of commission are actions taken that are not correct. Areas where risk is high is in the prescription of medications or conducting certain treatments.

Errors of Omission: Examples of errors of omission include cases where not enough or no treatment is given.

Inpatient Settings: Inpatient settings and inpatient care refer to care and treatment that is conducted within hospitals.

Malpractice Claims: Medical malpractice claims are those claims filed against a medical professional due to negligence by acts of omission or commission and that fall below the accepted standard of practice and have resulted in injury or death.

Outpatient Settings: Outpatient settings and outpatient care refer to care and treatment conducted outside the hospital and may include outpatient surgical centers, primary care offices, and outpatient specialty clinics.

PART II

CHOOSING PRIMARY HEALTH CARE PROVIDERS

- Who are the primary health care providers

- Criteria for selecting a good primary health care provider

- When to select a different provider

- Health care providers are human too: Nurture these relationships

CHAPTER 4

WHO ARE THE PRIMARY
HEALTH CARE
PROVIDERS

"America's health care system is in crisis precisely because we systematically neglect wellness and prevention."

Tom Harkin, United States Senator from Iowa since 1985 (Instrumental in Establishment of U.S. Office of Alternative Medicine in 1992, Born 1939)

WHAT YOU'LL FIND IN THIS CHAPTER:

- **DESCRIPTION OF THE ROLES OF THE KEY PROVIDERS WHO WILL DELIVER YOUR PRIMARY HEALTH CARE,**

- **CHOOSING THE APPROPRIATE PROVIDER FOR YOU,**

- **WHEN YOU DO NOT HAVE A REAL CHOICE OF PROVIDER**

Millions of new patients are entering the health care system with the implementation of current and future national health care reform. What kind of system and what kind of coordination of care are needed to deliver quality care to these individuals? A number of medical care specialists are involved in many aspects of patient care; however, we are focusing on the role of primary health care which is typically your gateway to the health care system. The primary health care system is critical to providing well care and prevention of illness.

ROLES OF PROVIDERS DELIVERING PRIMARY CARE

Primary health care providers see you literally, from "womb to tomb." These are the providers you are likely to see over long periods of time and are important to you because of the strong patient-provider trust that can be established. It is comforting to know that there is at least one health care provider that truly knows and is concerned about you and your family. Providers that deliver primary care can come from a variety of disciplines. They most often include family practice physicians, physician assistants, and nurse practitioners. In primary care offices you might also see and form a relationship with medical assistants who support the role of your primary care provider. The duties of each of these providers are determined by state licensure and often, national certification. We begin with the family practice physician.

FAMILY PRACTICE PHYSICIANS (FPPs)

FPPS represent that part of medical care devoted to comprehensive health care for people of all ages across genders, diseases, and parts of the body. These physicians treat patients in the context of the family and community, stressing disease prevention and health promotion. Treating an open wound and promoting proper diet and exercise might be addressed simultaneously by the family practice physician. These physicians provide care for a wide range of acute, chronic, and preventive medical care services. In addition to diagnosing and treating illness, they provide preventive care, routine checkups, health-risk assessments, immunization and screening tests, and personalized patient-centered counseling to achieve and maintain a healthy life style. In addition to family medicine, they may be certified in internal medicine, pediatrics, women's health, or gerontology.

For example, some FPPs might describe their practice with one or more of the following bulleted highlights:

- **TREATMENT OF ACUTE ILLNESS AND INJURIES:** for example, upper respiratory or urinary tract infections and breaks, cuts, and lacerations.

- **MANAGEMENT OF CHRONIC ILLNESS:** including hypothyroidism, diabetes, asthma, high blood pressure, and high cholesterol.

- **COMPLETE MEDICAL EXAMS:** for annual checkups and health reviews required by schools and employers.

- **CANCER SCREENING:** using U.S. Preventive Task Force recommendations for cancer screening of the breast, prostate, lung, colon, and skin cancers.

- **STRESS MANAGEMENT:** using holistic approaches with behavioral modification, relaxation, and mediation to treat everyday life stresses.

- **HOLISTIC ASSESSMENT AND HEALTH MANAGEMENT:** complementary and alternative therapies such as acupuncture, chiropractic care, homeopathy, massage therapy, naturopathy, and others are available through referrals.

- **MENTAL HEALTH AND SUBSTANCE ABUSE:** management of mental health issues and substance abuse prevention are available through referral sources and onsite nurse practitioner staff trained in assessment and short term follow up.

- **HEALTHY AGING:** treatment of conditions associated with aging, such as bone density, decreased levels of testosterone and estrogen, and decreased cognitive functioning (with referrals when needed). Education in healthy diet, exercise, sleep patterns, use of drug store nutritional supplements, vaccinations, and safety in the home.

- **WEIGHT LOSS MANAGEMENT:** combination of behavior change, exercise, and medications when needed to reduce weight and maintain weight loss.

- **PREGANCY AND POSTPARTUM CARE:** continuous prenatal health screening and postpartum management thereafter.

Note: While some family practice physicians will see infants, children and women during pregnancy, others will focus their practice on the care of adults, 18 years of age and older.

While this "menu" of service areas might not be available through a provider website, it is a good idea to discuss those that are important to you with your provider.

Another category of primary care physician is the Doctor of Osteopathy or DO. These providers focus on the whole-person approach to medicine and because of this frequently choose primary care, family practice, general internal medicine, or pediatrics. They make up a very small percentage of primary care providers. While the licenses are different, the medical training for the DO and MD are virtually identical. There is one exception; DO's are trained to manipulate the musculoskeletal system in an approach to diagnose and treat conditions like chronic headaches.

Today, many primary care physicians are open to alternative approaches to treating health conditions (e.g. chiropractic procedures, acupuncture, herbal therapies, and behavioral modification). Based upon their medical wisdom and patient preferences they may devise and carry out a treatment plan including these approaches or will refer patients to other community resources. Some of these procedures may be covered by your insurance plan but it will depend upon your condition, the state in which you reside, and the credentials of the provider treating you. For example, in Michigan you would be covered for chiropractic treatment; in California, for acupuncture; and in Oregon, neither of these therapies would be covered by your insurance plan. It depends upon what your state considers to be essential care.

NURSE PRACTITIONERS (NPS)

NPs are advanced practice nurses in positions to provide primary care in its entirety, and in many cases practice, independent from a supervising physician. They are fully trained clinicians that are likely to help fill the gap in the primary care workforce. With more physicians exiting their practice due to retirement or for other roles that minimize private practice administrative time and costs, NPs are and will be an important resource. NPs have received additional education and training beyond that of a registered nurse (RN). They can treat both physical and mental conditions performing most of the duties of physicians, but are frequently required to work under the supervision of a physician. They are able to take medical histories, make diagnoses, prescribe medications, and perform a limited number of medical procedures. They examine patients and formulate treatment plans. Often the treatment plan requires the NP to refer the patient to see the MD or a specialist.

There are several categories of NPs depending upon their specialty. For example, pediatric NPs and geriatric NPs work with patients of certain age groups. Family NPs are similar to family practice physicians and may treat patients of all age groups.

In some states NPs are required to work in collaboration or under the supervision of a physician. While NPs can prescribe medications in all 50 states, in some states they are required to have physicians co-sign a prescription and in some cases their subscription authority is restricted, such is the case with controlled substances. Controlled substance prescription use is monitored by the Drug Enforcement Agency (DEA) with the purpose of protection of the public against harmful use. They are potentially addictive drugs or drugs that could be abused by patients. Examples are: Cocaine for topical anesthetics, Morphine or Opioids, Ritalin used for treatment of Attention Deficit Disorder and several others.

The independent prescribing (prescriptive authority) of NPs is changing and with Federal Health Care Reform. In some instances they may prescribe without limitation, any controlled drug. Nursing organizations are seeking to achieve uniformity of state regulations in NP practice. With the implementation of the Affordable Care Act, these NPs will also have a broader scope of practice allowing them to practice independently from physicians. Many states are considering changes to existing laws to allow for the expansion of NP practice roles. In addition to NPs there are also other advanced practice nurses who are eligible to deliver primary care. These are Clinical Nurse Specialists.

PHYSICIAN ASSISTANTS (PAs)

PAs are often positioned to give care in primary care medical offices or clinics. All PAs are licensed. About half of all PAs are employed in physician offices. They can perform most of all the care physicians give, including taking histories, making diagnoses, prescribing medication, performing certain procedures. However, they must do so under the supervision of a physician. Supervision can vary; it may mean direct observation and supervision on a daily basis through on-site visits. Or, as in some rural areas where there are few physicians, this supervision may mean a doctor visiting once or twice a week to supervise the PA's practice. They may otherwise consult with a doctor only when they think necessary.

The education of PAs is similar to that of physicians, but can be completed in less time. Programs can be two or three years long and include clinical supervised training. Some programs grant Master's degrees, but this is quite variable since no award besides a certificate can be granted. PAs are allowed to prescribe only non-controlled medications. However, in some states they are required to have the co-signature of a physician or are restricted to prescribe controlled substances.

MEDICAL ASSISTANTS (MAs)

MAs are a fourth category of care provider but they are not considered to be primary care providers per se. They are however frequently found in primary care practice offices because they are there to assist. You may find them in an office along with both physicians and NPs. Typically, they have far less education than either FPPs or FNPs. Some may not have any formal training and learn on the job. Others may attend one-year certificate programs or two-year college programs awarding associates (AA) degrees. They may perform a variety of duties including those that keep the office running smoothly. For example, these duties might include monitoring insurance payments, scheduling appointments, or submitting insurance claims. They are also likely to perform clinical tasks, such as taking vital signs, preparing and maintaining examination and treatment areas, preparing patients for examinations, assisting with procedures and treatments, preparing and administering medications, health screenings and follow up of patients who have had laboratory tests. But be assured, these tasks should be performed in collaboration with the FPP or NP. No states require licensing of MAs. Still, many have received certification from programs offered by the American Association or Medical Assistants. Less than 15% of the MA workforce is certified. Approximately two-thirds of MAs work in medical offices. You will not likely see an MA working without a supervising physician or nurse practitioner.

CHOOSING THE APPROPRIATE PROVIDER FOR YOU

Choosing a provider is a process. This process includes several steps. Most importantly, you need to know what your insurance plan promotes or allows. You will need to reread several times the information your insurance policy provides you, particularly as it pertains to choice of practitioner and specialists and choice of treatment center or hospital in your area.

STEP 1: Carefully read your insurance documents.

STEP 2: You may want to ask members of your family, friends and/ or co-workers what they know about primary care providers in your area. This is especially helpful if you are new to the area. Hospitals close to you or university medical centers in your location may also give you helpful information about good primary care providers in the area.

STEP 3: By now you may have a list of names and locations. It is time to make a judgment about the credentials of these providers. Make sure all are licensed and certified. You can call the American Board of Medical Specialists to learn if your choices of physicians are board certified. For physicians, check your state's medical board's online website to identify whether there are any disciplinary actions or criminal charges filed against the provider.

STEP 4: Find out what affiliations your potential providers have with other treatment centers or hospitals in your area. To be affiliated with these centers or hospitals they will have had to meet specific quality guidelines. You may be able to determine whether any of your potential providers were refused privileges. This may or may not reveal a problem, but at least they are obligated to tell you why.

STEP 5: Double check to make sure your insurance plan recognizes these names and will accept them in your network. Also, check to make sure the treatment centers and hospitals the providers are affiliated with are covered by your insurance. It can be quite costly if they are not. Usually what happens is the insurance will fund your treatment by a non-approved provider at a lower cost than if it were in your network.

STEP 6: Find out if these providers have a home page on the internet. This page should list their credentials and even describe how they will cover your needs during non-working hours or while they are on vacation. Home pages are also an excellent source of information about their scope of service and whether the office staff are capable to perform the tests or treatments you need or whether they would refer you out to another primary care provider or specialist. For example, you may need a colonoscopy. These tests are performed every ten years primarily to detect colon cancer, but also to detect evidence of the development of polyps or growths in the lining of your large intestine. Will these providers refer you out or do they have the training and equipment to perform the colonoscopy in the examining room in their offices.

It is important to understand the providers' range of practice because if you are referred out for certain tests, screenings, or procedures other providers will be involved in your treatment plan. This means additional insurance claims and finding an office of someone you may never have seen before.

STEP 7: Make a visit. To buy the car you want you probably "shop around." In fact we shop around for many purchases. So, why not apply the same principles when choosing your primary care physician, office, or medical group? It is a far better idea to select on the basis of having researched and interviewed first. So what do you need to learn in a visit? Remember you have already asked trusted contacts, searched the internet for information and qualifications, and consulted your insurance plan. What is missing?

The answer to this question is "a lot." You don't yet know how the provider is likely to communicate with you, the professionalism of the office staff, and the pleasantness of the office setting. The provider must show you that trust and confidentiality are important. Could you trust the experience and knowledge of this provider? Would the provider have your best interests in mind? How strong are his/her communication skills, and how likely are you to be really listened to?

How professional is the staff? Are they courteous and friendly? Do they raise their voice with you? Do they talk about their personal lives (e.g. what a spouse said to them the night before)? Do they seem to run the office smoothly? Do they keep you informed about any delays in seeing your provider and reassure you? Do they reveal important details about you and your care within hearing distance of other patients waiting to be seen. If so, this is a violation of your confidentiality. If they are handling your medical account and billing, are they accurate? How pleasant are the surroundings? Is equipment and furniture clean and organized? Are left over specimens or test results left exposed? Are patient charts left open for view?

STEP 8: While you have collected necessary information to make your decision, one step remains: take the time to review the data you have collected and rank the providers you have seen. You may have already narrowed the search to one provider. This is fine, but remember to review each and every piece of information you have collected. This is also a good time to discuss your choice(s) with those who know you and you trust. At this point your choice is more clear and you will probably feel confident in making the best decision you can. Remember, this could be a lifetime commitment and it is well worth careful study to make this choice.

WHAT HAPPENS WHEN YOU DO NOT HAVE A REAL CHOICE OF PROVIDER

Current health care reform measures under certain circumstances will allow you to keep your current primary care provider if you have one. Additionally, you should be able to select a provider of your choice within your chosen network.

For those of you who are buying insurance through one of the new health care exchanges, it is possible that you will not be able to keep your provider under any of the plans available to you. However, you still will have a choice among the providers within the network you choose.

It is true that you will not be able to choose your own provider under all circumstances. If you have been covered under an insurance plan that does not meet the minimum requirements of health care reform then you will need to prepare to change plans and, most likely, provider. For those of you who get health insurance through an employer, things will pretty much stay the same. The exception would be if your employer changed insurance plans subjecting you to a whole new group of providers and provider groups.

Once you are a member of a group, you may be transferred to another provider within the group. It could happen that even though you chose a primary care physician, you may now be assigned to a physician assistant or nurse practitioner, or even a provider that just joined the group. This substitute may not have the expertise or "bedside manner" you prefer. You are expected to accept this arrangement and identify with the medical group, not the provider. Otherwise, you are a patient with canyon circle medical group, not a patient of Dr. Goldberg.

Also, if you need a procedure or test not performed in your current medical group, you will be referred to another physician or specialist who may be affiliated, but not within your current medical group. In fact, this provider may be some distance away from your home group.

Finally, if your provider retires or leaves the group you will automatically be reassigned to another provider. The new provider may be someone who you have never seen before. You may not be told in advance or asked about your preferences for the new provider. You may not have even been told about your provider's retirement or leaving the group.

These events are largely out of your direct control. You will be expected to stay in your original medical group. You may feel like turning to a different primary care medical provider group. This decision will have some repercussions. This may not be the best decision. It entails going back to the network to review all of the groups available to you. If you do feel this is the best decision, you will need to repeat the process (Steps 1-8) outlined for you in order to feel confident about the change to a different group or single provider.

Thus far we have addressed typical primary care available in most communities. The majority of you who apply for and receive affordable health care insurance will follow this route. There are alternatives we have not yet addressed. What if you decide to not choose a primary care provider and hence put yourself at jeopardy for not being able to access other medical services. First, many people have gone without identified primary care providers. The process is sometimes chaotic and not knowing who will see you and where to go is worrisome. Those without health care insurance and without a designated primary care provider or provider care group can still be seen. The options are free clinics or services that charge by scale according to what you can afford. County supported clinics and hospitals are an option. So are community health or mental health centers financed in part by the federal government. These services also charge on a sliding scale based upon your stated income. Another option is community free clinics. For example, women's health centers originally providing women's reproductive health care are now branching into provision of full service primary care.

A second alternative to be aware of are the increasing number of physicians working in the capacity of *concierge doctor. Concierge medicine (also referred to as retainer-based medicine)* is an arrangement between doctor and patient which offers stability for both. These doctors will usually take a smaller group of patients; for example, no more than 600 to 1,000 patients (the average annual caseload in primary care caseload can get as high as three times that number).

Concierge doctors remain with this same set of patients offering added accessibility and even in some cases, home visits. In turn, as a patient you would be expected to pay an annual fixed fee (which may vary widely by region from $195-$5,000) in addition to other costs of care such as medications, lab tests, hospitalizations, and emergency care. Some providers are on a cash-only basis whereas others accept insurance. The advantage of this kind of model is that the provider can keep overhead and administrative costs low while patients receive what has been assumed to be higher quality personalized care. There are no available data on the quality of care received at what cost. This model has been criticized for creating a two-tiered system that favors the affluent because those who can't afford it would not have the opportunity to benefit from any advantages it provides over the customary model of primary care.

The expected enormous increase in new patients entering the health care system in the next 6-10 years will cause changes in how primary care will be delivered and the choices available to individuals and families. While much is known there are still "gray" areas. It is critical that you are armed so that you know what may happen and how it will potentially impact you.

RESOURCES

1. Agency for Health care Research and Quality (AHRQ) http:// www.healthfinder.gov. An excellent overview of criteria to follow in choosing a provider along with specific questions to answer about the quality of care that might be available.

2. DocFinder: This website will help you find out whether a doctor you are considering is in good standing with the state board of medical licensure in your state.

3. *The American Board of Medical Specialties, Directory*: This resource can be found in many public or medical libraries and will tell you whether your physician(s) are board certified and what certification credentials they possess.

TERMS

Medical Assistants (MAs): Medical assistants are allowed to perform a variety of functions in primary care. These duties are in keeping with a more limited training program. They could include monitoring insurance payments, scheduling appointments, or submitting insurance claims. MAs are also likely to perform clinical tasks, e.g. taking vital signs, preparing and maintaining examination and treatment areas, preparing patients for examinations, assisting with procedures and treatments, preparing and administering medications, health screenings and follow up of patients who have had laboratory tests. These tasks must be performed in collaboration with the FPP or NP.

Nurse Practitioners (NPs): Nurse practitioners can perform most of the responsibilities of the primary care physician, including taking health histories, conducting physical examinations, making diagnoses, and performing certain medical procedures. They can also prescribe medications but in some states this duty may need oversight from a physician. In some but not all states NPs are allowed to work under little if any supervision of a physician. This privilege is controversial in several states, e.g. California, where physicians seek to retain oversight of their practice.

Physician Assistants (PAs): Physician assistants often give care in primary care medical offices or clinics. All PAs are licensed. They can perform most of all the care physicians give, including taking histories, making diagnoses, prescribing medication, and performing certain procedures. However, they must do so under the supervision of a physician.

Primary Care Physicians (PCPs) or Family Practice Physicians (FPPs): Primary care or family practice physicians are devoted to comprehensive health care for people of all ages across all ages, genders, diseases, and parts of the body. These physicians treat patients in the context of the family and community, stressing disease prevention and health promotion. They provide care for a wide range of acute, chronic, and preventive medical care services. They may function in private practice or group practice settings where they work collaboratively with NPs and PAs.

Primary Health Care Providers: Primary Health Care Provider is a generic term used to describe a variety of professional practitioners licensed and/or certified to deliver care in primary health care settings. While these practitioners (physicians and advanced practice nurses) can be found in inpatient health care settings, they are mostly found in outpatient settings. Outpatient settings are facilities where patients are assessed and treated but do not stay overnight. They can include surgical centers, specialty clinics, and private or group medical practices.

CHAPTER 5

CRITERIA FOR SELECTING A GOOD PRIMARY CARE PROVIDER

"The physician should not treat the disease but the patient who is suffering from it."

Moses Maimonides
(Physician and Scholar, Middle Ages)

WHAT YOU'LL FIND IN THIS CHAPTER:

- **WHAT ARE PRIMARY HEALTH CARE PROVIDERS AUTHORIZED TO DO**

- **WHAT STANDARDS ARE THEY HELD TO**

- **WHO ARE THE GOOD PROVIDERS ACCORDING TO PATIENTS**

- **WHO ARE GOOD PROVIDERS ACCORDING TO EXPERTS**

- **HOW TO CHOOSE A PRIMARY HEALTH CARE PROVIDER**

Good primary care providers are those with excellent diagnostic skills, the ability to teach you sound health maintenance and disease prevention self-care practices, and can manage your health conditions over time. Above all, they have people skills sufficient to engage you in a positive collaborative relationship. When selecting your provider you will also want to know not only the traits of the provider but the characteristics and efficiency of their practice setting.

Choosing such an important health care provider or doctor is difficult. If you have moved to a new community and have no idea how to find the best provider or doctor it is even more challenging. Ordinarily, you might ask someone (friends, family, co-workers, neighbors), but ultimately you are in charge of making the decision so you want to be as thorough as possible. Having to make that decision when you are sick is not ideal. It is highly recommended that you do your homework early on.

Your search will depend upon your needs and accessibility to providers in your community and your health care insurance program. Many people do not yet have a primary care provider, this is the first place to start. Your options to identify a specialist, if you need one, will depend upon whether and what kind of specialist your primary care provider thinks is needed.

As explained in Chapter 4, your insurance plan may restrict your choice of a physician or specialist. In this case you would be asked to choose from a group of plan-approved physicians or offer financial incentives to use plan-affiliated doctors. Always cross-check the terms of your insurance coverage to find out whether your plan will cover visits to the physician you are considering. Call your plan representative with the names and they will be able to tell you which physicians qualify under plan and will recommend a general or specialist physician.

WHAT ARE PRIMARY HEALTH CARE PROVIDERS AUTHORIZED TO DO

Primary care providers are the number one work force to serve the needs of our citizens. In fact, the largest portion of the care Americans receive is outside the hospital by these primary care providers. In the previous chapter, we detailed for you who these primary care providers were. We defined their roles and included medical assistants because you are likely to see this health provider in many primary care offices.

As previously detailed, physicians, physician assistants, and nurse practitioners make up the bulk of these providers. Internists and family physicians are the largest groups of primary care doctors for adults. These providers are equipped to give you care for most concerns you have, such as common conditions like a cold, the flu, or minor injury as well as annual checkups. Additionally, many women see obstetricians/gynecologists for some or all of their primary care needs. And, pediatricians and family practitioners are primary care doctors for many children.

As a review, we will touch on some very important points. There are limits on what physician assistants, nurse practitioners, and certified nurse midwives can do. Physician assistants, for example, must practice in partnership with doctors. Nurse practitioners and certified nurse midwives are authorized to work independently in some states but not others. Primary care providers, alone or in conjunction with nurse practitioners or physician assistants, are trained to take care of you for most of your health care needs and medical care. They are interested in helping you stay healthy but will also help you manage illnesses of longer duration over the long run. They are also prepared to refer you to a specialist (e.g. oncologist, surgeon, dermatologist, gerontologist) who treats specific conditions and who is an expert in diagnosing certain illnesses.

What Standards Are They Held To

Every licensed provider is fully credentialed to give primary care. This goes also for nurse practitioners and physician assistants. They have graduated from accredited university or college programs recognized by state boards of medicine or nursing. In the case of nurse practitioners, they are also certified by national credential organizations that oversee the quality and safety of the programs.

All health care providers are required to practice according to best practices and are forever bound by the Hippocratic Oath:

...and above all, to do no harm...

Every licensed health care provider must complete hours of training required by the respective State Board of Licensure to update proof of competence. The number of hours required differs by profession and state.

Who Are The Good Providers According To Patients

Several surveys of patients' opinions have been conducted over the years to identify what "good" and "not so good" providers have in common. Good health care providers, including doctors, are not only those that practice competently, they possess certain qualities that most patients value. Patients want to be understood as "whole persons," not just a disease. They want to be assured that their doctor knows a lot technically but are masters at applying this knowledge with skill and are able to relate to them as people capable of understanding their disease and its treatment.

To illustrate patients' desire for respect and humanness, consider the following survey. The results of a 2001-2002 study conducted by the Mayo Clinic patients reported their views of an ideal doctor.[1] Patients were asked to describe their best and worst experiences with a physician in the Mayo Clinic system. The interviewers independently identified

7 ideal behaviors. Listed here in no particular order of importance, the ideal physician is:

- Confident

- Empathetic

- Humane

- Personal

- Forthright

- Respectful

- Thorough

Further explanation of these characteristics revealed the following patient thoughts:

- Confident: "The doctor's confidence gives me confidence."

- Empathetic: "The doctor tries to understand what I am feeling and experiencing, physically and emotionally, and communicates that understanding to me."

- Humane: "The doctor is caring, compassionate, and kind."

- Personal: "The doctor is interested in me more than just as a patient, interacts with me, and remembers me as an individual."

- Forthright: "The doctor tells me what I need to know in plain language and in a forthright manner."

- Respectful: "The doctor takes my input seriously and works with me."

- Thorough: "The doctor is conscientious and persistent."

The authors noted that these traits covered doctors' behavior, not technical know-how. This is due most likely to the fact that patients feel more able to judge the interpersonal skills of doctors. Patients may assume that all practicing physicians are technically competent. Dr. Li who works in the allergic diseases division of the Mayo Clinic's medical school in Rochester, Minnesota drafted a list of opposites that might represent the characteristics of "bad" doctors in a survey of this kind. They include:

- Timid

- Uncaring

- Misleading

- Cold

- Callous

- Disrespectful, and

- Hurried

There are several sources of information that can help you evaluate your list of doctors by credentials and safety. The specific training, education, and certifications of doctors as well as disciplinary actions taken by the State Board regulating their practice in the state or states in which the doctor is practicing can be accessed through reputable web sites.

Other things to consider when choosing a primary care provider include the following (the answer to these questions might help you decide);

- Accessibility: Where is the practice located? Will it be easy for you to get there? Is it accessible by public transportation? Is there ample parking?
- Which hospital(s) does the provider use? Are you comfortable with the possibility of being treated at one of these institutions should the need arise?

- Where are routine x-rays and laboratory studies performed? Can these be done in-office or will you have to go to an outside laboratory?
- How long must you wait for an appointment after you call? Can you be seen on the same day if you have an urgent need? Is the office staff professional, friendly, and courteous?
- If you call with a question about your care, does the provider return your call promptly?
- Who covers for the provider when he/she is away? Whom should you call if you have a problem after-hours? If the provider works in a group, are you comfortable with being seen by one of the group practice partners?
- Does the provider frequently refer patients to specialists or does he/she prefer to manage the majority of your care themselves?
- Does the office process insurance claims, or must you pay up-front for services and file the claims yourself?

If you still aren't sure, ask if you can have an "interview" appointment to speak with the physician about your concerns. You may have to pay a co-payment or other fee for this service, but it can be a valuable way to gather information when making your decisions.

WHO ARE GOOD PROVIDERS ACCORDING TO EXPERTS

Experts in medical care have studied and analyzed what constitutes a good doctor.[2] These characteristics are similar to what you might think patients would say, but there are differences. They are summarized as such, "a good doctor":

- Leaves his/her personal feelings aside and doesn't let personal feelings bias care.
- Lets you fully explain your story or concerns.

- Manages time wisely so that the focus is on you.
- Communicates clearly and sensitively.
- Is clinically competent.
- Avoids common errors in thinking.
- Balances action with inaction (watch waiting).
- Makes recommendations warranted by your needs and not for financial or other personal gain.
- Is comfortable with uncertainty.
- Doesn't label your condition as some rare condition; it is likely that it is a common condition and this should be explored thoroughly.

How To Choose A Primary Health Care Provider

If you are already a member of a major health care plan or HMO or Health Maintenance Organization (e.g. Kaiser Permanente or the Veterans' Administration health centers) your choices will be controlled by the hiring practices of the HMO. That is, you are limited to those PHPs and doctors practicing in that plan. In that case you are relying on the plan to hire and monitor their doctors and other primary care providers for quality care. (*Note:* You have some choice within the plan to choose and change providers.)

If your health plan is not an HMO and covers the services of many providers, your decisions are critical to getting you the best care possible. It is important to be careful in your selection process. Why? Because there is wide variation in the quality of doctors and health care providers just as there is variation in quality of hospitals in America.

When checking on the doctor's experience and training, you need to know if he/she has experience with conditions like yours. Those with special training and a lot of experience are more likely to be an expert in the field and will be able to give you the highest quality of care.

There are several things you want to ask or know. The Agency for Health care Research and Quality (AHRQ) provides the following list when looking for a doctor. These are contained in the synopsis below; the doctor:

- Is recognized and rated to give quality care
- Has the training and experience in medicine to your needs for diagnosis and treatment
- Takes steps to prevent illness-for example, talks to you about losing weight, quitting smoking, getting adequate exercise, those things we know promote and preserve your health
- Has privileges at the hospital of your choice (has permission at the hospital to admit and treat patients in the particular hospital of your choice)
- Is part of your health plan (e.g. managed health care plan or health maintenance organization), unless you can afford to pay extra for care that would not be covered by your plan
- Encourages and welcomes you to ask questions about your condition and care
- Listens to you when you are describing your symptoms and the steps you took on your own to resolve them
- Explains things clearly and waits to assess if you understood them correctly
- Treats you with respect

AHRQ provides an excellent approach to help you apply these guidelines; for example, when checking the quality of the provider's practice you also want to know who did the ratings and if they are reliable. If there are reports from previous patients listed on the provider's web page you might question whether these remarks are really reflective of the provider's practice.

In conclusion, choosing a primary care provider is one of the most important decisions you will make. It may be that you will have this provider for an extended period of time. Many patients have the same provider for well over 8 years. Your choice might influence the choice of provider in your family and may follow through generations. Your decision rests on a number of things including your needs and accessibility to providers in your community and to a health care insurance program that will allow you to choose the provider you prefer. Additionally, your choice of a specialist, if you need one, will depend upon whether and what kind of specialist your primary care provider thinks is needed and one he/she respects. Because the choosing a primary care provider is a very important selection process it is imperative that you take time to consider all those qualities that make for a good provider as identified by others, patients like yourself and experts in the field of health care. In the next chapter the characteristics of a good and bad provider will be discussed in detail.

REFERENCES

1. Bendapudi NM, Berry L, et al. Patients' Perspectives on Ideal Physician Behaviors; March 2006. Available from Mayo Clinic Proceedings, 81, 3. Accessed November 3, 2013.

2. Gage, M. 10 Signs and Symptoms of a Good Doctor, Part 1 & 2; March 24, 2010. Available from: Whole Life: Cancer Coaching & Resources. Accessed January 9, 2013.

3. AHRQ, U.S. Department of Health and Human Services, Archive: Choosing a Doctor. Available at: www.ahrq.gov. Accessed November 3, 2013.

RESOURCES

There are several sources of information that can help you evaluate your list of doctors by credentials and safety. The specific training education and certification of doctors as well as disciplinary actions taken by the State Board regulating practice in the state or states in which the doctor is practicing can be accessed through reputable web sites.

- AHRQ, U.S. Department of Health and Human Services, Archive: Choosing a Doctor. Available at: www.ahrq.gov. Accessed November 3, 2013.

- Groopman J. How Doctors Think. Boston, Massachusetts: Houghton Mifflin Co.; 2007. This New York Times Best Seller by Dr. Groopman describes the workings of the mind of the physician and gives a clear portrayal of the important relationship between doctors and their patients. He reveals why some providers succeed and others make errors. He illustrates how providers, specifically doctors, can gain help from patients to avoid poor decision-making and poor communication with patients which eventually impact the level of quality care.

There are a number of online sites that have been shown to be useful. Among these are:

DocFinder.com: This website will help you find out whether a doctor you are considering is in good standing with the board of medical licensure in your state.

Healthgrades.com: Healthgrades is an independent company with a nationwide data base for rating the quality of doctors, dentists, and hospitals. It allows you to search and compare physicians by specialty, dentists, surgeons and other providers within in certain geographical areas. It also assists in making first appointments. It also assists in comparing the quality of hospitals in your area based upon three dimensions: patient safety, patient experience, and quality of clinical service.

Vitals.com: Vitals is a website that not only enables you to locate a physician by specialty, your condition, insurance plan, and your locale but will inform you about who you will or should see, what to expect, what questions to bring with you, what the diagnostic workup will be, and typical treatments or therapies that may be appropriate for you.

Vitals also rates physicians by considering four different points of view: peer ratings and awards, patient ratings, factual information about the doctor's expertise and academic background, and the office and office staff. Patient ratings are averaged on the basis of ratings 1-4 on the following indicators:

- Overall opinion

- Ease in getting an appointment

- Waiting time during a visit

- Courtesy and professionalism of office staff

- Accuracy in diagnosing a problem

- Bedside manner (caring)

- Spending enough time with me

- Following up as needed after my visit

Vitals also assist in making appointments online.

Whenever you are using independent rating websites it is important to evaluate the accuracy and quality of their data and conclusions. Evaluations and critical reviews of these websites are also published online.

TERMS

Accessibility: accessibility is the feature of being available to you. Historically, accessibility to primary health care has been denied to many. Health care reform through affordable health care makes obtaining an appropriate primary care provider significantly more possible. Still, there are other reasons this care may not be easily accessible. One clear challenge is how near this care is to you.

Affordability: affordability is the idea that health care is within your means to access. Under health care reform, insurance plans are required to cover you for basic preventive services. Insurance companies are also forbidden to drop you because of a previous illness.

Autonomy: autonomy is the characteristic of being free to select the provider of your choice without undue pressure to choose from a select few. Given the challenge to provide care to millions of new patients in the context of insufficient numbers of providers, autonomy in selecting the primary care provider of your choice may be limited.

Figure 1: Summary of What to Look for As You Choose a Primary Health Care Provider

You are looking for a provider who:

- Is rated by peers to give quality care

- Has no alarming patient reviews on internet sites

- Has the specific training and experience to meet your specific health care needs

- Is a provider within your insurance network (unless you can afford to pay extra outside your network)

- Has hospital admitting privileges or can refer you to another provider with hospital admitting privileges within your network

- Has good listening and relationship building skills

- Encourages you to ask questions and explains things clearly

- Takes time to teach you how to prevent illness and injury and manage your current medical conditions

- Treats you and your family with respect under all circumstances

- Protects the privacy of your records and personal information

Figure 2. How to Evaluate a Primary Health Care Provider During an Office Visit

After you have made a list of the primary health care providers or doctors most likely to help you think about making a visit to interview them. During this visit you will learn very important aspects that might influence how you would be treated especially how this provider builds relationships with potential patients. Many of these behaviors refer to the provider's "bedside manner." After the visit complete this form to rate the various aspects of the visit.

DID THE PROVIDER?	YES	NO
Show me respect?		
Make me feel comfortable?		
Ask me questions and encourage me to tell my story?		
Listen to me and the questions I had?		
Give me time to ask questions?		
Answer in terms and language I could understand?		
Focus on the problem or condition I came with or had questions about?		
Ask me what I already knew or had been told about my condition or health problem?		
Ask me what I already knew or had been told about the treatment of my condition or health problem?		
Ask me if I had preferences about different kinds of treatments?		
Explain his/her credentials and areas of specialization to help me understand his areas and levels of expertise?		

Note: These criteria may have varying importance to you. However, if you can't reply "yes" to 85% of the items there is a good indication that you would be making a mistake if you selected this provider or provider group. You'll want to trust your reactions but also know that the answers to these questions are not entirely predictive of the relationship you build together. It often takes several visits to recognize character traits.

CHAPTER 6

WHEN TO SELECT A DIFFERENT PROVIDER

"Whenever a doctor cannot do good, he must be kept from doing harm."

**Hippocrates of Cos (Hippocrates II)
(Greek Physician and Scientist, Regarded as the
Father of Medicine,
460-377 BC)**

WHAT YOU'LL FIND IN THIS CHAPTER:

- **WHEN TO CHANGE PROVIDERS**

- **DESCRIPTION OF TRAITS OF "NOT SO GOOD AND BAD PROVIDERS"**

- **PATIENTS REPORT BAD BEHAVIOR**

- **SELECTING ANOTHER PROVIDER**

Like so many of you, my family and I have been recipients of both "good" and "bad" care, all the better to understand what you are up against. I am drawing on a wide variety of observations and experiences to provide you useful guidance in not only managing the quality of your care but in understanding when it is time to change providers. This chapter is not about seeking referrals. Referrals usually come from your provider or from other institutions or specialists that you find or are suggested to you.

There may be times when you are searching for a provider or when you think about who you are seeing and conclude: "…not everything is negative _but_ I have enough information to tell me who this doctor really is as a person and physician and I want to move on".

As previously explained in Chapter 5, choosing a good primary health care provider or doctor can take some time and effort on your part. In this chapter reasons to think about choosing another provider, not just simply how to locate a provider and apply general criteria in your selection, will be addressed. What is a not so good and a bad provider will be discussed. There are some subjective criteria that will help you decide, but also some experiences along the way that will convince you that you are doing the right thing by changing your provider.

WHEN TO CHANGE PROVIDERS

The easiest way to answer this question is to review the needs and preferences you identified earlier. For example, if the provider does seem to have basic technical skills but treats you unkindly or has questionable standards of care, it is time to look for someone new. If you have done a good job with your initial search, you have most likely discovered a misfit through visits or initial treatments that were not handled ethnically or technically correct. Presented with the idea that you may need to change providers may be frustrating and you may worry, "what now?" Some group practices do not allow for you to change within their group and may tell you that it is your desire to change to another provider within the group you may have to go to a different medical practice.

Do not be shy about this step to make sure you get the best care possible. Some patients may feel that they are "traitors," especially if their initial relationship was friendly and supportive. It may become even more complex if the provider attends the same church, their kids attend the same school, or they work together. Regardless, "stick to your guns." This could be a matter of injury or even death to you. Hopefully, this discovery happens early and not after a medical error has occurred where you have experienced a medical injury. Since this is such a serious change you might be helped by knowing what providers are particularly problematic. In the next section of this chapter we will address what a not so good and a bad provider is.

DESCRIPTION OF TRAITS IN A "NOT SO GOOD AND BAD PROVIDER"

There are differences between "not so good providers" and "bad providers". "Not so good providers" may commit acts of omission or commission but these acts are far less dangerous. (See Chapter 3 for an explanation of omission and commission errors.) "Not so good providers" are categorized as such because they may lack certain skills or knowledge, but they do not go as far as to commit illegal or criminal acts.

In Chapter 5, we presented the traits believed by other providers to be exemplary of good doctors. In the Mayo Clinic survey of patient opinions, traits covered doctors' behavior, not the technical know-how.[1] The researchers thought that this was due most likely to the fact patients feel more able to judge the interpersonal skills of doctors. When listing the personal competencies of doctors, they also drafted a list of opposites that might represent the characteristics of a "not so good doctor." As you might recall, the terms used to describe a not so good doctor were personality traits, such as cold, callous, hurried and disrespectful. You can ask yourself, if the provider acts like this, what are the chances I'll really get the kind of care I want and that is of high quality?

It can be worse. You find yourself not with a good provider, not with a "not so good provider", but with a "bad provider", or more aptly put, a provider behaving very badly. Bad providers are clearly those who commit criminal acts. Borderline cases would be those providers through medical negligence killed a patient. Examples of extreme cases would be: a provider who killed patients by lethal injection or fatal poisoning. Other criminal acts that have cited in the literature and received public notoriety are those providers who have sex with an incompetent patient or one under general anesthesia. Perhaps less severe but still unethical and illegal are those providers who use, possess, or distribute controlled dangerous substances and drugs. Still others may commit Medicare or Medicaid fraud or practice without a license. Income tax evasion, fraud, bribery, or forgery and falsifying medical records have been linked to providers. Providers have also been convicted of DUIs and public drunkenness, but these infractions are regarded as less important provided the impaired behavior does not occur during a time of giving care or doing surgery.

There are several agencies that protect the public from "bad providers" and providers doing bad acts. A list of some agencies and how they function are contained in the resource section of this chapter. In its Principles of Medical Ethics, the American Medical Association (AMA) states that physicians shall respect the law and members should report physicians deficient in character or competence, or those who are known or thought to be engaging in fraud or deception. Membership in AMA can be denied to physicians convicted of criminal activity.

Patients Report Complaints: How To Process These Complaints

Some providers request patient feedback and openly listen to how their practice can be improved. Others do not. If individual providers do not seek evaluations from their patients it may mean that they don't need to because their large health care organization collects their evaluations as a matter of judging how well their organization is doing. Thus, the provider's performance is evaluated, but it might be the organization who is collecting the data.

AHRQ provides an excellent approach to help you gauge the quality of provider behaviors as posted. For example, when checking the strengths of the provider's practice you also want to know when the reviews were done and how many ratings were provided. It is also important to evaluate the credibility of the review. The issue is how valid and reliable are any of these ratings and whether they should impact your decision making. Reports from previous patients that are listed on the provider's web page might call into question whether these remarks are really reflective of the provider's practice or are biased one way or another: either too positive or too negative.

Still it is important to study the likelihood of their possibility and consider whether they are a deal-breaker for you. Some may be. The contents and believability are critical. For example, you read a negative review about a doctor in which the patient complained. But, you do not know what this doctor would say about the patient or the situation. Additionally, this negative statement does not reflect the strengths of the provider, particularly his/her clinical skills. Clinical skills are extremely important in the practice of primary care.

To determine whether this review is biased you will want to consider other comments about this provider and his/her staff. Are there complementary remarks? If these remarks praise the provider for being an excellent diagnostician, this is important. You will also want to know how this provider scores on any rating scale. For example, if the rating is 4.5 out of 5 with 25 reviews, it may indicate added strength because this rating would be interpreted as "very good" and the sample is decent for internet data of this kind. Still, you don't know how representative this group of reviews are (the annual average caseload a primary care physician's practice can be as high as 260 or more). Only 25 reviews out of 260+ patients posting reviews should be viewed cautiously. And you don't know whether these reviews are biased in any way because of the manner in which such reviews are obtained. Overall, there is evidence to suggest that the provider is a good practitioner despite a negative remark by one patient. Your trusted friends and advisors may provide you with additional data and perspective.

Here is an example of another patient's remark about a different provider: "I have been very impressed with Dr. (X's) attention to detail and willingness to take the time to listen during my treatment visits... He is the first physician ever that...completely understood what I have been going through, took the time to listen, and offered a great treatment plan. His level of caring is very high..." These remarks are very positive and communication skills are very important to you. You are likely to respond positively to this provider and put your trust in his/her practice.

SELECTING ANOTHER PROVIDER

It is not entirely known how many patients leave a provider without reporting a near mishap or an incident of borderline or flagrant criminal behavior. What is known is that these events happen and perhaps more often than you might guess. It is unknown at what stage in their treatment patients leave. Are their conditions fully assessed? Are they in the middle of a complex therapy or treatment program? Are they more likely to stick it out than move on no matter what?

We need patient "whistle blowers". There is a new program in the works to tap into what patients know about medical errors and unsafe provider care. In the past there was no widespread formalized way to collect this data. The Agency of Health care Research and Quality is looking to encourage patients and their families to report using a website and in telephone interviews.

But let's go back to the issue here: how are you to select a different provider? Sometimes the process is one of getting a second opinion. You seek or you are recommended to go to a second provider practice. Starting this process is like the one you went through initially in choosing a provider, but depends a lot what has happened for you to mistrust your provider and what is going on with your health. If time is on your side, you will review and update your list of needs and preferences. It is not just a matter of selecting a different provider within the provider group. Some practices do not allow for you to change within their group and may tell you that if that is your choice you will have to go to a different medical practice. Your provider network and insurance plan will help you with this process. Call your plan representative and they will be able to recommend an alternative based upon your needs for a general or specialist physician.

Hopefully, you have not suffered a medical injury, but if you have you or someone close to you will need to act quickly. If you are not able to get to a second doctor right away this may be a case of going directly to a hospital emergency room or urgent care center.

In either case, **DO and I mean DO** immediately seek another primary care provider practice and a second opinion. Remember, you are the employer, the insurance plan pays your employee, and you are entitled to fire your doctor or provider at any time. When you do change, make sure that you obtain a copy of your medical records from your treating provider's office.

REFERENCES

1. Bendapudi NM, Berry LL. et al. Patients' Perspectives on Ideal Physician Behaviors; March 2006. Available from: Mayo Clinic Proceedings, 81(3): 338-344.

RESOURCES

- The American Medical Association. AMA collects data about how safe physicians are in their practice,

- The Administrators in Medicine web site provides information about disciplinary actions or even criminal charges filed against physicians in your state,

- Selected states obtain and report malpractice information, this would include practicing without a license, and

- Local Boards of Health are able to make malpractice information available publicly.

TERMS

Medical Negligence: Medical negligence is a term frequently used in medical malpractice claims. It is one aspect of the claim. It may refer to the failure to act by a provider when, under standards of care, there was clear cause to do so. Otherwise, this would be an omission error. This term is found in legal cases to establish the basis on which fault occurred. Negligence may not always lead to a malpractice claim; but, when it leads to patient injury or death it is a good case for medical malpractice.

Patient Whistle-Blower: Patients and patients' families have a wealth of information about medical errors and unsafe provider practices. By reporting what you experienced and observed you are fulfilling an important role as a whistle-blower.

CHAPTER 7

HEALTH CARE PROVIDERS ARE HUMAN TOO: NURTURE THESE RELATIONSHIPS

"Health care providers owe you their time and expertise.... not their lives...."

The Author

WHAT YOU'LL FIND IN THIS CHAPTER:

- **HEALTH PROVIDERS WANT A COLLABORATIVE RELATIONSHIP**

- **STRESSES AFFECTING YOUR PROVIDER**

- **ARE YOU ANNOYING OR MAKING YOUR PROVIDER UPSET**

- **HOW TO REPAIR YOUR RELATIONSHIP WITH YOUR PROVIDER**

Providers are humans too. This means they experience joy and pride in their work, but also are at risk for worry, stress, and frustration. These are just a few feelings among other responses to their work environment, life's rewards, and disappointments. Although educated to leave personal problems aside and do their best to form good interpersonal relationships with each and every patient, their intentions may not always work as planned. You can help your helper!

Good relationships with your health providers rest not only with how your provider treats you, but your behavior as well. Don 't forget they are human too! They get stressed, they get sick, they can love what they do, they worry about their families....and the list goes on. The intent of this chapter is to give you insight into the inner workings of what it takes to work in the health care world from a provider's point of view and how that might impact your relationships with them.

HEALTH PROVIDERS WANT A COLLABORATIVE RELATIONSHIP

Health providers understand that helping patients is dependent on having a good working relationship. The foundation of this relationship is a two-way partnership based upon mutual respect and trust. If such a relationship exists patients are likely to experience safe and quality health care. To establish a collaborative relationship the patient must feel empowered to actively participate in exploring health concerns and to make informed health care decisions.

Research has shown that the most impressive improvements in chronic disease management are probably due to interventions specifically designed to enhance patients' abilities to manage their care in active collaboration with their providers. For these reasons active involvement is important to you.

Some patients interpret this to mean that they need to become just as informed as their provider. They may search the internet researching symptoms, diseases, and the latest treatments. What they lack is the professional judgment and experience of the provider. Never assume you can make important health care decisions without collaborating with your provider. This includes: diagnosing your condition, choosing among several treatment options, altering the prescribed treatment, and terminating your care without consulting your provider.

STRESSORS AFFECTING YOUR HEALTH PROVIDERS

Health providers experience stress on a daily basis. Sometimes the stress is extreme and is influenced by the number of emergency and traumatic conditions they witness. Death and dying can be particularly difficult to face on a constant basis. Additionally, treating medical conditions may be hurtful.

Infectious disease and accidents on the job (e.g. exposure to lethal toxins) can threaten their own lives. Violent patients or those that are unusually difficult to manage add to their stress. Can you imagine an AIDS patient threatening to "spit in your eye" or a patient biting you or throwing something at you? These things happen.

Add the pressures of having to treat too many patients with too little time to deliver the best care possible, day in and day out, the situation can result in the *professional stress syndrome* or *burnout*. Such conditions are widely reported among all categories of providers, even early in one's career.

The stress providers experience might seem to them to be endless and not easily avoided. Even when providers take good care of their own mental and physical health, stress is always present and the consequences can be serious. The stress of upcoming changes in health care delivery can take their toll as well. This is especially so if these changes mean longer work hours to treat many more patients. Providers may begin to feel that they have lost their professional autonomy and don't have enough time to deliver the care to which they are committed.

All in all, loss of control over their practice is a critical concern and one of the biggest contributors to feelings of burnout. Loss of control over how many patients they see, how much time they have with them, how many different conditions these patients exhibit, and pressures to release patients from care or the hospital early are just some examples. Plans are to treat millions of previously uninsured patients may mean increased stress and burnout to providers.

Yes, providers have and may think about leaving their professions and will most likely try to change the circumstances of their practice, for example, to take fewer patients. Still, with increased pressure, some doctors might feel that early retirement is the only answer.

The ability to change practice conditions is unrealistic for the bulk of providers and will be in the future. No matter how well trained they are, how organized they are, no matter how committed they are to quality care, they are going to face high levels of stress.

ARE YOU ANNOYING OR MAKING YOUR PROVIDER UPSET OR ANGRY?

Just as some doctors lack interpersonal skills, patients may also do things that annoy or upset providers. Sometimes patients are unaware of these infringements. Let's take a look at very common patient behaviors that are upsetting to providers. Usually they can be categorized as: lack of respect, withholding or hiding problems, lying, being uncooperative, and not following the provider's advice or treatment plan.

Disrespect: What fits in the category of lack of respect? There are many examples of this. First, there are rude and obnoxious responses. Most likely this is due to their anger at the provider or some aspect of their illness or care. Other examples include not paying attention or refusing to answer questions, and being continuously late for appointments. Sometimes patients will promise to pay the bill or to submit forms to insurance companies for payment, but do not. You can imagine that if you went to a friend and borrowed money and said, "I will pay later..." and failed to do so, keeping that friendship intact is unlikely.

Lying or hiding problems: Secondly, patients may tell out right lies about their condition or what they are doing to treat themselves. Providers need to know everything related to a potential diagnosis and choice of treatment. Lying or hiding important facts can delay understanding your condition and even make your problem more difficult to treat. Also, you may not explain up front the reasons you are making the medical visit. Leaving out important information only hurts you and your care.

Being Uncooperative: Being uncooperative includes collecting important information to properly diagnose and treat you. You may do a poor job at describing your symptoms. This is excusable, but if the provider teaches you how to collect data and you fail to follow directions, your provider will think you are being uncooperative. Not bringing reports, medical records, or x-ray results when you were instructed to can also be viewed as lack of cooperation. Not sharing your expectations for your visit or care can be viewed as lack of cooperation. If you have certain expectations, such as getting a specific medication, the best thing you can do is say so. Your provider may not agree, but at least you are entering into a collaboration and encouraging a discussion about why. Leaving the visit without asking the questions you have is also not fulfilling the steps of being cooperative. Even if you sense that the provider is rushed and may not have the time, ask them anyway. Your doctor can tell you briefly, assign the nurse to explain it, or defer the discussion until your next visit.

If your provider suggests a particular treatment and you do not want this treatment or medication, say so. Nodding your head or saying nothing leads your provider to think you will follow directions. Taking a prescription form and failing to fill it, or fill it and then throw the medication away or just store it, will not help. If the provider suggests a medication, but after going to the pharmacist you find it is too expensive, call your provider and explain. There are usually other suitable medications.

If you are afraid of medications or afraid of the one you are asked to take, don't worry about what your provider might say, discuss it with him/her. Not complying with the treatment that your provider has chosen is a big mistake. The reason may have something to do with fear or the fact that you were not fully consulted about side effects or other issues. If you do not go back and explain your feelings, but continue not complying your provider may mistakenly think that it was the medication or treatment that failed, not you.

HOW DO YOU REPAIR YOUR RELATIONSHIP WITH YOUR PROVIDER

What if you did do these things, but didn't realize their consequences and didn't intend to jeopardize your relationship? Some of these actions can be corrected and communications repaired. However this is not true for all. Misleading and being untruthful is one of those not easily excused. Disrespect may not. Failing to adhere to the treatment plan may. In this case, all is not lost. Consider these steps to repair your relationship *faux pas*.

1. Think about what caused the problem. Were you forgetful or afraid of the treatment? Did you think it would cause serious side effects or effect your functioning in ways you couldn't afford? Were you afraid to discuss this with your provider?

2. If possible, make an appointment to discuss the problem. If it is a matter of not paying your bill, make a plan with your provider to pay down the amount. If you failed to follow the treatment plan then a full discussion and answer meeting is needed. In this case the provider may help resolve some of your fears or help to adapt the plan more to your lifestyle. If you (have been/are) influenced by the research you have done on the internet then bring this information along and share it.

3. If you have corrected the problem it is still wise to convince your provider that they are the best one to care for you, and that you will discuss all barriers to following a treatment plan with them in advance and with their input. Based upon your provider's response you will know whether the relationship has been repaired enough to continue to provide you high quality care.

4. If you are not able to repair the relationship and you think the result is far below par, then it is time to change and look for a different provider. While doctors are professional and have abilities to develop insight and compassion, this will not always be the case. Remember, providers are human too! It is better for you to direct your energies towards finding a new provider and establish a positive relationship, using the lessons you've learned.

In summary, the goal of any health provider-patient relationship should be one of mutual respect and trust based upon collaboration. Work together with your provider to achieve the best medical outcomes. Most of the time this is what happens. However, sometimes the relationship gets out of kilter and either you both repair the relationship as soon as possible, or you must be prepared to move on and establish such a relationship with a new provider.

REFERENCES

1. Shanafelt TD, Boone S, Litjen T, et al. Burnout and satisfaction with work life balance among US physicians relative to the general US population. *ARCH INTERN MED.* 2012; 172(18):1377-1385.

2. Dyrbye L N, Shanafelt TD. Physician burnout: a potential threat to successful health care reform. *JAMA*, 2011; 305(19): 2009-2010.

TERMS

Collaborative Patient-Provider Relationship: A collaborative patient-provider relationship is a partnership in which patient and provider are working together with a similar understanding of the patient's needs and goals.

Burnout or Professional Stress Syndromes: Burnout or professional stress syndromes refer to a combination of stress symptoms that can impair a provider's performance and ability to form a therapeutic alliance with patients. It can decrease quality patient care, lead to increased risk of medical errors, and increase provider job turnover.

PART III

SKILLS TO WORK COLLABORATIVELY WITH YOUR PRIMARY CARE PROVIDER

- Communicating successfully with your health care provider

- Managing your health care and treatment effectively

- Keeping your health care records and coordinating your care

CHAPTER 8

COMMUNICATING SUCCESSFULLY WITH YOUR HEALTH CARE PROVIDERS

Patient Addressing the Provider: "What you [Provider] want to know is not in the answer to your question, but I [Patient] will answer it anyway."

Anonymous Patient (1994)

WHAT YOU'LL FIND IN THIS CHAPTER:

- **COLLABORATION WITH YOUR PROVIDER REQUIRES EFFECTIVE COMMUNICATION**

- **PRINCIPLES OF COMMUNICATION AND YOUR ROLE IN EFFECTIVELY COMMUNICATING**

- **HOW YOU CAN HELP REDUCE ERRORS BY SHAPING AND RESHAPING YOUR DISCUSSIONS WITH PROVIDERS**

- **USEFUL TOOLS YOU'LL WANT TO USE OVER AND OVER**

There is no doubt about it. The quality of your care is directly linked to how effective your communication is with your providers. Without good communication between you and your provider not even adequate care can be provided. Further, whatever difficulties that do exist can result in harm to you in the way of errors of omission and commission. You may be at risk for increased pain and injury, added disability, and even early mortality. It is not an issue of being dissatisfied with the level of communication; rather, just what results from poor communication.

In this chapter, you will be introduced to some basic principles of communication that apply widely, but are also very important in relationships with your primary care providers. Effective communications are at the core of your getting quality health care and it would seem that this is easy to get. Unfortunately, this is not as easy as it would seem to be, or you would hope it to be.

COLLABORATION WITH YOUR PROVIDERS REQUIRES EFFECTIVE COMMUNICATION

Throughout this book your role as an active participant in your care is stressed. You have the right and responsibility to participate actively in your care. Your active participation is fostered by your knowledge and skill in communicating with your providers. You, your family, and your provider need to communicate as often as possible and effectively. In both instances this means perceiving appropriately, learning the language and symbols used in each one's culture, correcting communications that are ineffective, and sorting out and eliminating confusion and environmental interferences.

There are a number of communication skills your provider should bring to discussions with you. They include:

- Respectfulness and readiness to communicate
- Ability to actively listen to your story and what concerns you
- Ability to talk to you in language you will understand

- Show empathy and understanding when you describe aspects of your health difficult for you to manage
- Ability to address miscommunication in a patient and respectful manner

In turn, you are expected to bring certain communication skills to your visits in order to ensure effective communication and collaboration with your providers. Some of these are actually the same as those the provider brings to the meeting. These include:

- Respectfulness and readiness to communicate.
- Know in advance what questions you have and provide a list if useful.
- Ability to explain as concisely as possible what concerns you and what you want to know.
- Willingness to ask for clarification about terms or words you don't understand.
- Ability to ask for explanations of what is next and what is the plan. Communications between you and your provider are some of the most useful and rewarding you will ever have. Both pro-viders and patients value them for what they learn and for the interpersonal closeness they offer.

Principles of Communication and Your Role in Effectively Communicating

Principles of communication explain how we send and receive messages to get what we want. An enormous amount of research has revealed important aspects of human communication; much of which is so commonplace we don't recognize that we operate within these guidelines each day with all relationships. There are principles of communication that are important for you to understand when actively participating in your care. They are the following:

- Communication has a function value.
- Communication is both verbal and nonverbal; you always communicate something.
- Communication is a feedback process: encoding, sending or transmission, receiving, processing (coding and decoding).

Let's take the first principle and apply it to your ability to effectively communicate with your providers: communication has a function or utility value. When you visit a primary care provider, you are using communication to serve a function. It is useful in describing what you are concerned about and what you need to hear back from your provider.

Several problems that commonly occur and which patients complain about are the following:

(1) Providers not really listening to them

(2) Feeling that providers haven't heard what is really important

(3) Not having enough time to fully explain what is important

(4) Having to repeat things over and over to different providers

These are barriers to the utility value of your communications. The more you try to correct for them, the greater the likelihood you will get your needs met and the greater your satisfaction with the visit. Your role is to be persistent in making your requests, persistent until you are satisfied with the feedback you receive.

The principle that one always communicates is also important to your understanding of your relationship with your providers. This means that even if no words are spoken, something is being communicated. Communication is both verbal and nonverbal. of the latest tests. Verbal is the messages being passed orally or in writing between you and your providers. They have content (e.g. "Are the results of my lab tests better?"). The content is about lab tests and the results. But there is another dimension: the nonverbal context of the communication. Let's take your nonverbal first. If you are worried about your tests, this worry will be displayed in your expressions and tone of your voice. The provider on the other hand will communicate to you using separate non-verbal messages (e.g. hopefulness or even mutual worry).

How are these feelings communicated back to you? First, they may be disguised. It isn't that the provider is trying to lie to you or even hide the severity of the test results. But this may be confusing because you can not read the provider's real opinion through the nonverbal responses. Your role is to clarify both the content of the message and the underly-ing meaning expressed in the provider's nonverbal clues. You can reply, "Ok, I get that the test results are ok for now, but I think you might have certain opinions or that you are worried about them too. Right?"

The last principle of communication is about the process of commu-nication and this gets us into ways communication can be effective or ineffective. You assemble data and formulate a question that combines all of what you heard. You have reduced this information to something you can ask your provider. This question may be about prostate can-cer (i.e. "Am I at risk for prostate cancer?"). You send or transmit this concern in the form of a comment and question to your provider: "My father was diagnosed with prostate cancer, do younger men get it?" This is a legitimate question, but unless you say: "Can I get it at this age?" or something else to this effect, your chances of getting the kind of consul-tation you want may be jeopardized. And, let's say that the provider was very busy and studying your chart instead of really looking at you or hearing the concern in your tone of voice, your concern may be missed. But, let's say your provider is astute and picked up on your nonverbal worry and tone of voice and addresses this issue. In fact, the provider decoded correctly what your need was. Something might go wrong here. While the provider decoded correctly, the next task is to encode and transmit a message back to you about what you said or asked.

Let's say the provider starts out fine, but veers into a related subject about lung cancer being a far more common cancer in men, and asks if you smoke. This is also good information and the provider is correct; however, it might be tangential to your concern. What is your role? If you did not get enough of the kind of information you were seeking you could bring the provider back to your topic. Otherwise, maybe you want to know if you should get prostate specific antigen (PSA) tests regularly.

The illustrations discussed are examples of what could occur and result in communication that is either effective or ineffective.

HELP REDUCE ERRORS BY SHAPING AND RESHAPING DISCUSSIONS WITH PROVIDERS

When you are being assessed by your provider, they are applying a stream of thought that leads to conclusions about what does or might ail you. This process is called "assessment" or "assessment and diagnosis". Communications in this stage are extremely important because if they are poor they may lead to errors, and these errors could have devastating consequences for you. You are going to need some background in this process to fully understand what this means.

There are several communication and thinking errors that have been detected in providers who make mistakes, particularly when they are interviewing you to take your health history and make a diagnosis of what is bothering you. One set of errors is referred to as the 3 A's. The A's stand for: Anchoring, Availability, and Attribution.

Anchoring refers to the tendency of the provider to a hang on one aspect of what you are telling them. A provider can anchor on a specific aspect of your history and rule out other factors that you reveal. Otherwise, the provider's mind pulls tricks and only processes what fits or confirms their original judgment.[1]

Availability is another pattern. With this pattern your providers are strongly influenced by the most alarming cases they have seen. These cases are more prominent in their memory. They remember them because they are unusual. When you describe your problems they begin to clump your descriptions into a package of symptoms that resemble these memories that are easy to recall. These may be the experiences with patients most recently seen.

Finally, *Attribution* refers to the case when your information fits within a preset conception of you, the person, rather than weighing all the data available. This error often occurs when you are being negatively stereotyped due to your age, race, religion, or educational background. An example of this kind of problem would be the provider who believes you are eating too much fast food because you are a member of a certain ethnic or cultural group. In this case, you would be negatively stereotyped. You could also be positively stereotyped and this would also hamper the diagnosis of your condition. Let's flip the scenario and say you were from a group that had nutritionally sound eating habits. In this instance your provider would ignore asking or even hearing your description of eating fast foods 5 nights of the week. The problem with attribution is that your provider must be open to a variety of ideas and being influenced by stereotypes will not help. In essence, it closes discussion before the diagnosis process is complete.

If you see these problems occurring you can correct them. In each case you may believe that your provider is listening openly to what you are saying. Your job is to check on these perceptions and offer up different ideas. What follows are specific descriptions of errors and how you might communicate to correct them.

THE ANCHORING ERROR:

You are explaining a pain you are having in your lower abdomen. You say you have had it for two weeks on and off and you are worried because there are ulcers in your family and you don't know if this could be a sign of your getting ulcers too. Your provider latches onto the idea of an ulcer as if taking a short cut rather than taking the time to consider multiple possibilities. You try to follow the provider's thinking and hope the answer will be "no, I don't think you have an ulcer."

STOP RIGHT HERE

What you really want is a full discussion of what the pain is about. If your provider has not done so already, disrupt the anchoring error and change the topic to any or all of the following:

1. What makes you think that it isn't?

2. What else might be causing these pains?

3. If it is one of these other possibilities, how will we make sure?

4. What else do we need to know?

THE AVAILABILITY ERROR:

Availability is another cognitive mistake and when you think it is happening you can reshape the discussion. Availability errors resemble anchoring errors because in both cases your provider is being distracted and influenced by recent exposure to patients that had similar conditions as yourself. This is the case where the provider may think you have a diagnosis that has appeared often. Your symptoms might resemble those in other patient cases, but in actuality they do not fit this pattern entirely. This mistake follows when a provider is acting too quickly or not taking the time to study your case in depth. You can slow the pace and pose questions to help you and your provider think more broadly:

1. What are those cases you have been seeing?

2. How are my symptoms similar to those that these people had?

3. What are the differences between my symptoms and those that these people had?

THE ATTRIBUTION ERROR:

You are talking to your provider about losing weight after a recent pregnancy. You come from a culture where being "big" is a sign of health and happiness, but you think differently and believe that if you could lose a few pounds it would make you feel "better". Your provider reassures you that the weight will drop off soon enough and that your husband probably is "enjoying" your full figure. You reply again that you would feel better if you lost some weight. Your provider tells you to come back in 3 weeks, and if you haven't lost a couple of pounds then we can talk about a plan.

STOP RIGHT HERE

What you may want is to discuss how you are feeling mood wise and you have a thought that losing weight might make you feel more at ease. Disrupting this error can be done by the following:

1. Explain that you think differently about being "big" and explain how it makes you feel.

2. Bring the topic back to what you are feeling, if you are feeling "down" or depressed and stressed, talk about it.

3. Ask questions about what feeling depressed is and whether it is usual to have these feelings.

4. Above all … ask what you can do about them in addition to a nutrition and exercise program.

USEFUL TOOLS YOU WILL WANT TO USE OVER AND OVER

In this discussion we will focus on techniques to enable you to more fully understand what your providers are saying or have told you.

The first is "the feedback loop". The feedback loop works like this: Your provider explains something to you, for example, how to lose weight. Several minutes go by and you hear some really good advice about supervised weight loss programs. You are even handed a pamphlet to read when you leave the office. The only thing is that in the discussion the provider has talked about points that you were previously unaware of and even some points that you previously didn't believe. What to do:

1. First, stop the provider in mid-conversation and report back what you heard (i.e., something like this: "You're saying that I should keep to 800 calories a day for a week....and that I could do this for up to 3-6 months...that's not what I have heard.... isn't it unhealthy to keep doing it for so long....can you tell me if I heard this right?")

2. Listen to what you are told and repeat back again if there is still something that is confusing to you.

Graphically, what has happened is that you and your providers have made a loop (hence feedback loop) where:

(a) They spoke.

(b) You reflected back what you heard.

(c) Your provider had the opportunity to clarify.

Perhaps the most frequently recommended technique to use when visiting a primary care provider is to bring a list. This will help you become an active participant in your care and decision-making about health issues. There are at least two types of lists. There are lists of your medical history and medications you are taking. There are also lists of questions you may have about your health and treatment.

Lists are critical for several reasons. First, the list encourages to think about and write down all those questions you have about your health and medical care. Second, a list completed prior to going to the office visit allows you time to get input from others and even search the internet about these issues. Your list is becoming more refined and maybe becoming even more informed. Third, when you bring your list to the visit you will be less able to forget something you wanted to ask. You have your list and you can write down the provider's answers as the discussion unfolds. Sometimes providers may ask for a copy of your list or the chance to read it over to make sure they didn't miss anything. You can even ask that a copy be placed in your medical file. So the *LIST* promotes effective communications.

In summary, in this chapter a number of issues about communications with health care providers have been discussed. The point was made that effective communications are a two-way-street. That is, both you and your provider need to bring communication skills to the table to ensure effective collaboration. In some cases you will bring a family member or advocate. Patient Advocates is a new discipline that has offered a great deal to patients and families when they are having trouble navigating through the health care system in matters of gaining access to care and dealing with financial issues. Some medical centers and hospitals have referrals to qualified advocates including those who speak languages other than English. There are also websites that identify and describe the role of the patient advocate and you are encouraged to read them. These individuals can serve as useful coaches to you, but remember the key to effective communication is forming that special interpersonal relationship with your provider that fosters trust and openness. Patient advocates know and understand the importance of acting on your behalf, but also encouraging the special relationship you can form with your provider.

In primary care, your provider may be the one trusted person that stays with you over time and even cares for the next generation of your children and grandchildren. You will want and deserve effective provider-patient communication which is the core of quality health care practice.

FIGURE 1. POTENTIAL PATIENT COMPLAINTS ABOUT COMMUNICATING WITH HEALTH CARE PROVIDERS:

- Having to tell my story over and over again.

- I can't understand what my provider tells me.

- Sometimes they tell me what to do. but don't write it down, so when I get home I'm confused.

- My provider uses words that I can't understand.

- I ask a question and get a non-answer.

- They are too busy to hear what I have to say or listen to me.

- Staff can be rude and disrespectful.

- My conversations get interrupted ....they have to leave the room...and sometimes not come back.

- I see different doctors/providers all the time. They don't seem to know what's going on....each one tells me something different.

REFERENCES

1. Groopman J. *How Doctors Think.* Boston, Ma.:Houghton Mifflin Co.; 2007.

RESOURCES

- Groopman J. How Doctors Think. Boston, Ma.:Houghton Mifflin Co.; 2007. This book is a New York Times Bestseller. This is an excellent resource for learning more about errors in diagnoses and covers the communication errors of anchoring, availability, and attribution in great depth.

- Palmieri P. Suffer the Children: Flaws, Foibles, Fallacies, and the Grave Shortcomings of the Medical Care of Children. Amazon (Kindle Edition); While this book focuses on the care of children it is very useful in understanding errors in thinking and communication in a variety of clinical settings. It also covers errors of anchoring, availability, and attribution but much more.

- Patient Advocate Foundation. www.npaf.org/. This website provides information about the organization, the role of patient advocate case managers in matters of medical debt, financial assistance, Medicare resources for seniors, Medicaid specific resources and applying for Social Security Disability. Providing medical advice is not within the scope of their services.

TERMS

Anchoring Error: Anchoring refers to the tendency of the provider to a hang on one aspect of what you are telling them which confirms their original judgment.

Availability Error: With this pattern of thinking the provider is strongly influenced by alarming cases they have seen. These cases are more prominent in their memory.

Attribution Error: In this case the provider has a preset conception of you and your behavior. Rather than weigh all available data to determine a specific and unique diagnosis stereotypes your behavior and thus your condition.

Empathy: Empathy is the process or capacity while communicating to be aware of, sensitive to, and understand someone's feelings, thoughts, and experiences without having experienced them.

Feedback Loop: The feedback loop is a way of clarifying what you heard and understood the provider to say or mean. It starts with them speaking to you, then you speak back by reflecting on what you heard and what you thought it meant, and lastly, your provider clarifies any misunderstanding or gap in understanding you might have.

CHAPTER 9

MANAGING YOUR HEALTH CARE
AND TREATMENT EFFECTIVELY

*"Laughter is the best medicine...unless of course, you are
really sick...then follow what your provider suggests."*

The Author

WHAT YOU'LL FIND IN THIS CHAPTER:

- **WHAT ARE YOUR RESPONSIBILITIES IN MANAGING YOUR HEALTH CARE**

- **MANAGING THE ASSESSMENT AND TREATMENT OF YOUR HEALTH AND MEDICAL CONDITIONS**

- **WHY TREATMENT ADHERENCE IS SO IMPORTANT**

Ever increasing trends in health care are under-foot to encourage you to be more active. This means being more aware of your health and functioning, making sound decisions, managing your care, and measuring whether treatments are helping or not. You are considered an important part of the health care team. You have the power to make or break the success of the care you receive. You are at the hub of the wheel influencing what happens. This is your rightful place. All services should revolve around you; not a provider, not a single service center nor hospital.

What Are Your Responsibilities In Managing Your Health Care

The importance of your responsibilities in managing your own health and medical care have long been recognized. Healthy life style promoting behaviors (e.g. reduction of stress, physical activity, good nutrition, and supportive environment, as well as spirituality) have been sited as protecting you from illness and injury. These factors are proven relevant over time and cross culturally. They are the important ingredients in maintaining health and caring for your own well-being. Still, when you become ill there are new sets of expectations that land on your shoulders and require you to partner with health care providers.

Self-management of your health care requires you to know and understand your responsibilities. You may not have given too much thought to what these might be; however, we ask you to give them serious consideration if you are going to master your health care in today's health care system. There are many statements of patient responsibilities. Health care programs and hospitals you select will generate a unique set of responsibilities. While they may differ to some degree, they are likely to include these roles. You are expected to:

- Fully participate in decisions involving your care and treatment.
- Know your rights and responsibilities.

- Explain your understanding of the care planned for you and what is expected of you during this care.
- Know your rights and responsibilities.
- Provide your health care providers with the most accurate and current information regarding your health and symptoms, and any past illnesses, hospitalizations, medications (including health supplements).
- Follow your providers' instructions, adhere to aspects of your treatment plan, including medication taking, procedures, and recording results of self-administered tests.
- If for whatever reason, you can not follow your health care providers' instructions, report this to your provider as soon as possible, and ask for clarification and advice about what to do next.
- When using medications or other treatments that may periodically run out, inform your providers in advance before none is left.
- Medical devices and prescriptions are for your use only, don't share these with others even though you may not use your entire supply.
- Provide written permission for release of your medical records.
- Keep your appointments; when unable to, notify health care providers within a reasonable amount of time so that other patients may be scheduled for care.
- Be responsible in paying copays and insurance coverage in a timely manner.
- Inform your providers of any changes in personal information so that your records can be updated appropriately; this includes changes in insurance coverage, name, phone, and address changes.
- Show respect and consideration to health providers and staff. Be aware that some abusive behaviors and contentious behavior may result in your dismissal as a patient.

MANAGING THE ASSESSMENT AND TREATMENT OF YOUR HEALTH AND MEDICAL CONDITIONS

In this section of the chapter, three important aspects of managing your health and medical care are addressed. They are: (1) Assessment, (2) Planning and Implementing, and (3) Evaluating your care.

(1) Assessment. Assessment of your health is a matter of applying all your senses and what you know about yourself to decide whether what it is you are experiencing is something *different*. When you do this you are identifying *symptoms*. Symptoms are what you, the patient, recognizes; your provider will investigate further. What you are experiencing might affect your functioning and/or cause you to worry. It is the answer to the provider's question: "What is bothering you?" "What can I help you with today?" You will answer with whatever words best describe your subjective experienced symptoms. This is where you tell your story.

Don't be surprised if your provider turns your description into something that is meaningful from a medical perspective. For example, you may describe what you are feeling as: *something is just not right*. Your provider might note that you are suffering *malaise*, a vague condition that might be associated with a variety of medical conditions.

Your provider will be helped if you can say what it is and how it is affecting you. There are a wide variety of symptoms, including: pain, abdominal discomfort, bleeding, fatigue, restlessness, sadness, stress, weight loss or gain, or blurry vision. Sometimes they present together (e.g. fatigue and thirst or stress and sadness).

Your provider will look for *signs* of disease or injury. Signs are what your provider detects after examining you, running laboratory tests or performing other diagnostic procedures. Sometimes your symptoms will also be the provider's signs. For example, bleeding is both a symptom and sign if it is detected by both you and your provider. However, pain is not since your provider has no real objective method of proving you are in pain or measuring the intensity of the pain you have.

The symptom of pain presents a key challenge to you; it is subjectively felt, but objectively largely undetectable. You must be very observant of this symptom. You'll want to describe it as best you can: what you are feeling and how it is affecting you. There are certain descriptive words that are helpful. For example, can you describe the intensity and quality of the pain you are experiencing? What is the location and nature of the pain; is the pain you are feeling dull, sharp or piercing, continuous or reoccurring? Can you rate the intensity, say on a scale of 1-10 (with 10 being most severe you have ever experienced)? How long have you had the pain, and has the pain changed over time, lessened or increased? When is your pain the worst and has it affected your sleep, eating, working, or any other daily functioning?

Any descriptions you can give your provider will make it easier to understand how you are subjectively experiencing the pain. The symptom of pain may be tricky because the location of the pain you report may not be the place of concern. For example, some pains are deferred. That is they may be experienced in your shoulder, neck, or back, but actually involve another part of your body (e.g. your chest in the case of an impending heart attack).

Your report and your provider's assessment using tests and procedures will allow your provider to make a *diagnosis*. A diagnosis is the process by which your provider, using all available information, decides the cause of your problem. Diagnoses help to focus in on what treatment is needed and how you will view your prognosis.

Prognosis is a prediction of the probable outcome of your disease or injury based upon your condition and observations of other cases where the same or similar treatments have been used. Prognoses can depend upon many things and therefore it is not always easy to answer patients' questions in this area. For example, in the case of cancer, important factors are the type and location of the tumor, the stage of the disease when first diagnosed, the extent to which the disease has spread to other parts of the body and where it has spread, and the cancer's grade or how abnormal the cancer cells appear under a microscope. This will give some indication of how quickly it will grow and spread, and therefore, how lethal it is. Other factors that influence a patient's prognosis are the patient's overall health, age, and extent to which the patient responds to available treatment.

(2) Planning and Implementing. Once a diagnosis is made, plans for and implementing a chosen treatment is next. This is a critical stage for you. It is imperative that you understand the plans and your trusted friends or family (if available) are there to understand and support your decision-making.

Of course your condition may be *nonlife* threatening (e.g. with a broken bone, urinary or respiratory infection) or your condition may be *more* threatening (e.g. with a chronic or acute life-threatening illness). The more threatening conditions are *serious chronic illnesses* and *chronic debilitating diseases. Chronic illnesses* include: heart disease, cancer, and stroke. *Chronic debilitating diseases* would be: Rheumatoid Arthritis (RA), Parkinson's Disorder, Multiple Sclerosis, Cystic Fibrosis, Chronic Obstructive Pulmonary Disease (COPD), Schizophrenia, Dementia and Alzheimer's, or Multiple Sclerosis.

Whatever your condition or health care issue, your provider will discuss the various treatment options available. This discussion will include the pro's and con's of all treatment or therapy options and any side effects you might experience from each of the chosen treatments. It is important that you understand as much as you can and bring helpful others to appointments to be clear about what your choices are and what are the best options. Once you have chosen a plan you will learn in more detail what treatment and therapy is involved. But this is best understood before you have made a choice. Many treatments are not set in stone and will require you to remain on the program for a period of time to determine the effectiveness of the chosen treatment.

(3) Evaluating Your Care. You are an important participant in evaluating the effectiveness of the care you receive. Evaluation requires you to use some standard against which you measure your progress. You will be evaluating your symptoms on the basis of whether they are increasing or declining. When concentrating on your symptoms, you want to apply the same criteria that you used in assessing these symptoms. Otherwise, the location, intensity, duration or frequency, and degree to which the symptom(s) impact your activities of living or daily functioning are key features.

For some symptoms, you can use a measurement scale. This approach might not be useful to or desirable for everyone but they are available if you are interested. Measurement scales are very useful in identifying changes in a variety of symptoms including respiratory (such as cough and congestion), fatigue (such as with arthritis), bleeding (such as in wound healing), and fever (such as in infectious disease). They are also available for measuring emotional symptoms, such as anxiety and depression. If you are measuring duration of the symptom you can build a weekly calendar and track how many days or what portion of the day you have the symptom. If it is an issue of intensity, you can chart intensity during a single day or over a 24-hour period by specifying intensity on a scale of 1-10 (with 10 representing the highest intensity you have experienced). You can keep these charts current for the entire time you are being treated using a specific treatment protocol or regimen.

This kind of record is valuable not only for you to reflect on your improvement, but also to your provider in gauging how well a treatment is working for you. Your provider will also compare the results of the treatment against how it should work given a specific medical standard and how it has worked with other patients having the same condition and set of symptoms.

Measurement scales can be found on websites, or your provider may offer you a form to help you track your symptoms. Examples of measurement scales are available online and through Foundations or National websites. For example, the Arthritis Impact Measurement Scales (AIMS) is available through the National Arthritis Foundation. This scale measures symptoms and functional impairment in elderly patients. Another important screener available online is the Center for

Epidemiologic Studies Depression Scale (CES-D) Disease Control – Depression inventory. It is used for helping people to determine if they are experiencing depression at a level needing further evaluation. It asks about depressive feelings and behaviors during the past week.

If you are not using any measurement charts or scales, it is still imperative that you devise some way to talk to your provider about the therapy you are using and participate actively in the evaluation of your care plan. When you do this you'll want to describe the character of your symptoms and what you have observed over time.

WHY *TREATMENT ADHERENCE* IS SO IMPORTANT

It is time to address a critical issue of your treatment: whether or not you follow the treatment plan the way it is intended. We call this *treatment adherence*.

There are thousands of treatments available to bring relief from illness and cure diseases. For these outcomes to occur you will need to follow what medical advice is given to you, assuming it is of high quality. Following this advice is referred to as being *adherent* to medical regimens.

Treatment adherence is rather simple to understand and it is important for you to know. The World Health Organization defines adherence as: "…the extent to which a person's behavior - taking medication, following a diet, and/or executing lifestyle changes, corresponds with agreed recommendations from a health care provider."[1] WHO's most recent publication on adherence stresses the point that: *"Adherence to therapies is a primary determinant of treatment success. Poor adherence attenuates optimum clinical benefits and therefore reduces the overall effectiveness of health systems"* (WHO, 2013).

On the contrary, failure to follow medical advice or non-adherence has resulted in suboptimal treatment, risk for relapse from illness, and poor quality of life. Non-adherence can be full non-adherence or partial non-adherence. For example, you might not do anything your provider tells you to do.

Take, for example, managing diabetes. Self-management of diabetes frequently includes glycemic control (controlling blood sugar levels) through diet, medication, and exercise. It requires you to monitor your blood glucose level on a daily basis, which with today's technology is very easy. Still you could fail to follow all instructions. In the case of full non-adherence you wouldn't take your medications, follow any of the provider's advice about diet and exercise and, wouldn't self-monitor your blood glucose level. This would be called full non-adherence because you failed to follow everything you were instructed to do.

Partial adherence would mean you might take your medications, but not carefully monitor your blood glucose levels at the intervals you needed. Partial adherence may not have the same negative consequences as full non-adherence, but it could significantly impact your health and well-being over time and eventually cause worsening of your diabetic disease.

The quality of your communications with your providers is directly related to your adherence to any treatment plan. Can you believe this: patients can and do ignore what their provider advises and still continue making appointments for regular visits. There are good and bad parts to this behavior. First, it is good that the patient is returning to see the provider at all. This will give the provider the opportunity to detect the problem and the chance for the patient to discuss it when the provider asks. Providers can do very little for those patients that chronically ignore their advice and fail to discuss their concerns. Also, you are more likely to follow the medical regimen your provider has given you if you disclose your concerns, understand your providers' description of your condition and treatment options, and understand how to modify your behaviors, ask questions, and carry on a dialogue about how you could adopt any directions to your individual life style.

Information about your medications might be found on the internet and you might act upon what you read. Or, you might ask family members who are taking the same treatment about what to do. Some people ask the available pharmacist. Remember that it is still important to talk to your provider about your concerns. Some providers will answer questions like these through e-mails provided they know you well and were the ones to prescribe the treatment or medication.

There are several types of adherence that are relevant; they include whether you:

- Return for treatment and follow up (referred to as persistence in adhering to the medical plan).
- Fill medication prescriptions.
- Take medications as prescribed.
- Follow the providers' directions about improving your health and preventing complication or worsening your existing illnesses.

The maximal benefits from any treatment plan will not be achieved if you discontinue interventions before completion of the treatment. Disengaging from treatment or dropping out are serious and can limit overall effectiveness of the treatment. This does not mean you shouldn't stop your treatment if something is wrong or the treatment makes you feel worse. If this happens, you want to stop the treatment and call your provider as soon as possible.

A special case of poor adherence is medication non-adherence. We know that medications do not work if you don't take them, right? We also know that over half our population under age 64 is taking some medication; this increases to over 90% for persons 65 and over. In the treatment of all major chronic illnesses (arthritis, asthma, hypertension, major psychiatric illness, diabetes, pulmonary disease) adherence to medication regimens is concerning because these illnesses by themselves or in combination require many medications.

All of us are at risk for poor adherence, but patterns of non-adherence have been studied. For example, it is documented that patients do better just before an office visit (white-coat adherence) and worse when they tire of the demands of the regimen (e.g. 18 months after starting the medication). Also, patients pick and choose which medications out of several they might follow more exactly. Reasons for not taking a selected medication are numerous and include fear of side effects, embarrassment, simply forgetting, failing to fill a prescription, and attitudes about the medication prescribed. For example, some people don't take their antidepressant medications because they feel embarrassed or ashamed of their condition. They may even believe they are not depressed to avoid letting others know that they are being treated for depression. This could be missed by the provider if the patient has been adherent to taking other medications.

Patients do not adhere equally across all medications. These observable phenomena suggest that it is important to be aware of your own patterns of becoming non-adherent and to track your adherent behavior in an attempt to prevent serious non-adherence. It is possible that your adherence will wax and wane over time because no one can be 100% adherent.

Many patients use medication adherence tools. These are daily pill boxes, refrigerator magnets, or even timers. In addition to tracking your medication taking behavior, it is also important to examine what happens when you are prescribed new medications. Although your provider may describe the medication, the need for it, how to take it and what to do if you have problems, things still can go wrong.

First, you may not know exactly what to observe and what to report. Prescription medication packets always have a drug insert and your local pharmacy can explain certain things to you. In fact, it is always important to talk to the pharmacist and make sure he/she knows all the medications you are taking and verifies that the mix of drugs is safe. Still you may be unclear. Do you decide:

(1) Take the medication anyway.

(2) Call the provider's office and wait for a return message.

(3) Take some portion of the medication (some is better than none).

(4) Call someone else and ask them, maybe they have taken this medication before.

(5) Look up the medication online and take what is said to be the average dose.

(6) Do nothing until the next scheduled provider visit.

(7) Go see another provider and see whether this new provider will prescribe the same medication.

(8) Some combination of all the above. The best step to take is to call your provider and report what you are experiencing and your concerns. Never let your provider be uncertain that you are taking your medication.

In conclusion, more than ever before you are being asked to take an active role in managing your health and any treatment you are getting. You are not alone in this process. Your health care providers are by your side. However, working collaboratively and cooperatively with them can make all the difference in the world in your recovery and ability to secure your highest quality of life.

REFERENCES

1. World Health Organization. *Adherence to Long-Term Therapy: Evidence for Action*. Available at: www.who.int/chp/knowledge. publications. Accessed November 4, 2013.

RESOURCES

Resources include several measurement scales helpful to you if you have one or more chronic illnesses. They focus on measurement of symptoms.

- National Arthritis Foundation: Arthritis Impact Measurement Scales (AIMS)

- Visual Analog Scale (VAS). This scale helps you chart your experience of pain by asking you to place an X at the point on a scale that best represents your experience of pain.

- Center for Epidemiological Studies- Depression Scale (CES-D). This 20 question inventory can be found online and is a commonly used measure to evaluate depressive symptoms. It can be self-administered and scored online. You will also be guided in determining your level of depressive symptoms based upon your which is calculated for you. You can take the results of your inventory to your provider to discuss the need for further evaluation of depression.

TERMS

Adherence: Adherence is the extent to which a patient's behavior in following medical recommendations does or does not follow the recommendations of the health care provider.

Non-Adherence: Non-adherence refers to not following recommendations of the provider.

Partial Adherence: Partial adherence refers to following some directions, but not recommendations.

Full Adherence: Full adherence refers to following all or close to all recommendations in the manner the provider recommends.

Daily Functioning or Activities of Daily Living (ADLs): These are basic activities of people and include self-care functions (e.g. feeding, bathing, dressing, grooming, working or exercising, and rest and relaxation). When we experience symptoms they sometimes impact how well we can perform these basis human functions.

Diagnosis: A diagnosis is the process by which your provider, using all available information, decides the cause of your problem. Diagnoses help to focus in on what treatment is needed and how you will view your prognosis.

Managing Care (Phases of Assessment, Planning, Evaluating): You have a role in several facets of your health care management and treatment. The first phase is *Assessment* where you observe your condition and note any changes or concerns that occur. These symptoms, sometimes very vague experiences need to be discussed with your provider. The second phase is *Planning and Implementing* and follows the diagnosis of your condition. It is a process of mutually deciding on what your options are and committing to a course of action. In this phase you are instrumental in following your plan in the manner your provider recommends and reporting back whether there are any problems with the plan. The third phase is *Evaluation*. In the evaluation phase you are collecting evidence about the progress of your treatment plan. This may include charting any changes in your symptoms, such as whether they are subsiding. This information along with your providers observations help determine the extent to which your care and treatment are successful.

Prognosis: Prognosis is a prediction of the probable outcome of your disease or injury based upon your condition and observations of other cases where the same or similar treatments have been used.

Self-management: Self-management refers to your ability to manage your own care. It includes any strengths or deficits you have in performing the phases of assessment, planning and implementing, and evaluating your course of treatment or therapy.

Symptoms and Signs: Symptoms are those changes you observe and are felt subjectively by you which means that others may not be able to detect them unless through your own self-report. Signs are those clues observable by your provider and are collected through a physical exam, blood tests, x-rays, or other diagnostic procedures.

CHAPTER 10

KEEPING YOUR HEALTH CARE RECORDS AND COORDINATING YOUR CARE

"With tens of thousands of patients dying every year from preventable medical errors, it is imperative that we embrace available technologies and drastically improve the way medical records are handled and processed."

Jon Porter, former Congressman from Nevada Third Congressional District (Born 1955)
[http://www.brainyquote.com/quotes/keywords/medical_records.
html#CfWAMYs0I6QI3F2X.99]

WHAT YOU'LL FIND IN THIS CHAPTER:

- QUALITY CARE IS DEPENDENT UPON YOUR CARE BEING COORDINATED

- TOOLS TO ENSURE YOUR CARE IS COORDINATED HOW YOU CAN PROTECT THE PRIVACY OF DELICATE INFORMATION

Making sure your health care is coordinated is very important. It makes a great deal of difference to safe delivery of health and medical care. Coordinated care provides a system of communication channels in which all persons involved in your care are familiar with and communicate about your medical records or conditions. There are several tools in place to make coordinated care happen, but you have a significant role in seeing to it that every health care provider knows all there is to know about your health and medical care.

Quality Care Is Dependent Upon Your Care Being Coordinated

With the successful implementation of health care reform all U.S. citizens should have access to a large range of health care services and these services will increase in numbers through time. With an increase in services there is a greater need for coordination. The question is how best to track these health care experiences and how will you communicate them to all who should know your health history. Coordinated care refers to having communication links between services across all aspects of care, from your primary care giver to your physician in a specified field.

Coordination between health care providers involved in your health care is particularly critical during transitions between sites of care, such as when you are being discharged from the hospital. Failure of treatment can occur due to the fact that one set of providers is poorly informed about the opinions and directions of the other treatment sites.

Tools Available To Ensure Your Care Is Appropriately Coordinated

Maintaining thorough records of the medical care you receive and exercising oversight over your records are two ways to ensure that your care is up to date and that the information is complete. Medical records provide a complete list of your medical history, physical exams, lab test results, tests/procedures you have had done, and treatments you have received. You will have a medical chart at all of the offices, clinics, and hospitals that treated you over the years.

Medical records can be stored on paper or electronically. The recommended method is electronic. Electronic Medical Records are not new; they have been in existence since the 1960's. Growing attention has been placed upon them in the Government's attempt to reform health care and provide people equal access to quality care. Millions of prescriptions and medical reports are now computerized and are part of the new health care reform agenda.

Health and medical records that can be easily transported from one provider to another are key to ensuring coordinated care. The most common records for improving channels of communication are: Electronic Health Records (EHRs) and the Electronic Medical Records (EMRs). Still another format is the Personal Health Record (PHR) that some of you may already keep. All of these forms of records can be help coordinate care if they are shared and discussed across providers.

1. Electronic Health Records (EHRs): are centralized databases containing a collective and comprehensive medical history and related information that can be shared across different health care systems. Because they provide the opportunity for channeling communication to different providers they are helpful in achieving coordinated care. These records include a variety of health related information from many health professionals including your primary care providers, hospitals, and clinic services. They can be extremely helpful in coordinating your care because they tell the provider exactly what records to retrieve and where to get them. Additionally, they alert providers to who should receive copies of information about the care you are receiving currently. The exact mechanisms for use and deployment with new health care reform is yet to be finalized on a wide scale.

2. Electronic Medical Records (EMRs): are similar to EHRs and play a significant role in coordinating your care, but they are records from a single provider. Many, but not all, providers use EMRs today. You will find that your primary provider or provider groups use them. Data from this single provider is electronically collected, monitored, stored, and maintained in the provider's office.

EMRs also differ from EHRs in that they are generally less comprehensive because they are limited to the care provided to you by a single provider or provider group. In other words, information from your hospitalization and visits to specialists do not appear except in the form of a summary. What are absent are the specific details of the treatment course or tests you underwent. Should your provider want these specific details, it is possible to get them. When obtained they would be included in your provider's electronic medical file. Remember with EMRs you can have numerous files because each of your providers will have their own set of electronic files on you and your care.

3) Personal Health Records (PHRs): Unlike either EHRs or EMRs, a PHR is a record with information about your health that you, or someone helping you, keeps (this form of health record is also described on the website: Medicare.gov). PHR includes the following information:

- Your basic information:
  - Name
  - Birth date
  - Address
  - Phone number
  - Emergency contact information
- Your Personal Information:
  - Marital status

- Religious affiliation

- Place of employment

- Your Medical Information:

  - Family history of chronic/life threatening illnesses

  - Last physical examination performed and the name of the provider who performed it

  - Current list of active medications and treatments (this includes the doses of the medication and when it was prescribed)

  - List of allergies you may have to certain medications

  - List of any supplements or over-the-counter drugs you take

  - A complete list of major illnesses and surgeries (including the name of the doctor and the date of the procedure)

  - List of infections and injuries and treatment plan (include who treated you and when)

  - Results of the most recent lab tests and screenings (e.g. EKG, EEG, or MRI) and dates of tests/screenings

- Your insurance information:

  - Health care insurance plan

  - The name of all the providers who are currently treating you (this includes their name, phone number and address)

Although something like this could be kept in a folder or written file, increasingly these records are kept secure with different internet programs that you can adapt for your personal use. PHR programs give you a unique user ID and password, giving you control over who sees it (even your providers will not be able to access it without your permission). Most information that is in your EMR can be downloaded to your PHR. Some providers and hospitals will offer you a way to view your medical records and download the information to your own PHR.

Your PHR will keep all of your health information in one place. This makes it easier for you to find information about both past medical services and recent health care. You can build a chronological list of services and changes in your treatment plan if you are being seen and followed for a chronic illness. Data in a PHR can help providers get the information they need in case of emergencies. It is good to provide your emergency contacts with a copy of your PHR in the case that they may need to provide this information to the police or emergency medical technicians.

The format of this information is important because you want to make sure it is easily read and retrieved. You can use a variety of sources to find a PHR format. Some providers and health plans offer them for free. There are also independent vendors that create and maintain PHRs. Some will actually create and maintain your PHR for you if you give them your permission to access your health information from your health plan and providers. Medicare.org recommends the site: myPHR. com Globe icon as a source. AARP offers a PHR tool free to its members. This format has a number of helpful tabs (e.g. for medications, health conditions, allergies, insurance); you can enter as much or as little information as you choose. The U.S. Surgeon General's Office is still another source for a personalized health record. This tool is a family health history record (My Family Health Portrait) that can be shared with other family members and your health care provider. It is free and also open to everyone. All of these options have procedures to protect your information from unauthorized access or use.

In selected advanced medical centers there may be an elaborate electronic system that performs a wide range of information that will be helpful in keeping updated health records. This information is electronically entered and stored online and includes not only their account of your health information but lab results and graph trends of your lab findings. It also provides you the opportunity to message your provider, refill a current medication, request an appointment or referral, and find information about a previous visit and upcoming appointments. There is no charge for this service. You can pay your bill online through this service, find a provider, and read about research and clinical trials at the center. It is confidential and allows you to access the information any time and any place. Unlike emailing your provider, it uses secure technology and only you and your provider (or provider's authorized staff) have access to your patient portal.

In sum, the use of EHRs, EMRs, and PHRs combined are tools both you and your provider use to keep an updated account of your care. These tools facilitate coordinated care and with providers using this information your condition and treatment are likely to be known to all those caring for you even though they could be miles apart.

In addition to keeping an updated account of your care, you have another role in fostering coordination of your care through a health record. This role is one of oversight. This means keeping track of what is in your PHR but also how well your records coincide with those of others. While providers will be able to track issues with your care and detect some lack of accuracy, you are needed as well.

Checking how well your records match others is important. However, there is another particularly important step: watching out for discrepancies in the listing of treatments or medications you are taking. Specifically, you are looking to see if the entries are identical. In the case of medications, does your list match what providers think you are taking? Your provider's list, for whatever reasons may be invalid. Check the medication names, doses, when they were prescribed, and if they were discontinued. The number of errors in medication lists are significant and common. The kinds of discrepancies may include:

- Medications that are current versus those that have been discontinued

- Dates medications were modified and what modifications were made
- When new medications were added or discontinued

It is not usually the route of administration (such as by mouth orally or by injection) that is confused, but the dose and whether other medications were added or deleted. There can also be a discrepancy if you decided on your own to delete a medication or add something without discussing it with your provider. This is how your record can inform your provider about how you are managing your own care. You may be making a serious error that could have negative effects on your health. If this happens you need to discuss the discrepancy with your provider right away.

Any changes you make in your PHR would reflect your provider's decision to change what you are currently doing. This opportunity is a good one because it reinforces that your care is a collaborative process. In a perfect world we would find there to be no discrepancies and would expect our providers to be on top of these types of errors. But, we are working in a health care system that is over burdened with data and many more patients than we can easily track.

Validating with patients what they are taking and doing is recommended when there is a transition in your care (e.g. going from home to hospital or hospital to home). At this time it is likely that new medications might be ordered or existing medications are rewritten. The aim is to create the most complete and accurate profile of your current treatments and medications and compare them to what your own medical records say. The reason why this is done is to avoid medication errors, such as: omissions, duplications, drug interactions, or dosing inaccuracies.

To help you perform the task of checking how well your treatment and medication list matches your provider's, there are medication reconciliation forms. These forms actually perform a coordinated care function which is to discover important discrepancies between you and your providers. Like PHRs, there are vendors who make these forms and encourage you to use them rather than construct your own. The form is usually a chart that allows you to keep all current information at your fingertips. They allow you and your family to keep a current list of all pertinent medical care information, including your immunizations, allergies, prescribed medications, and supplements you are taking. You can find them online and download a form that you favor. They are simple to complete, but first you want to gather as much paper evidence as you can. Let the form guide you by filling in the blanks. For example, list all your medications including the providers who prescribed them.

You can keep the information in written form but it is better if you can download and type the information so there is no confusion. Now you are ready to print your form and take it with you to visits with your provider, or trips to hospitals or clinics. You always want to keep the form up-dated because it is the one form that will be useful in reconciling what the providers know about you and what is actually the case. It is even wise to save the form to a flash drive and keep it with you at all times.

How You Can Protect The Privacy Of Delicate Information

There are several ways you can protect the privacy of your electronic health records. Special permission from you, or passwords that you select known only to those you permit to view your records, are effective. You will also want to be sure the website is secure; vendors that offer PHRs have secure websites to protect anyone from breaking in and accessing your data without your permission.

Other important regulations about the disclosure of your health information that you need to know about are contained in HIPAA privacy regulations.[1] You should be informed about HIPAA regulations during your medical visits. You will be provided a list of the policies and will be asked to sign and date that you have read and understand your rights and protections. They are in full implementation and have significant implications for how your providers handle your information and your rights to access your own records. They allow you to see your medical records, request corrections, and obtain documentation of disclosures of this information. Under these policies you should be able to find out who has requested information and what was shared with them.

HIPAA rules regulate how your provider or health care systems protect your information when coordinating your care. Infractions carry penalties if your providers and insurance company violate policy. For example, insurance companies and employers can be penalized if your privacy rights are violated. These penalties may include fines as well as criminal charges. It also requires each organization (e.g. medical office, clinic or hospital) to set up procedures to protect your privacy when transmitting your information to other health care agencies.

In summary, the process of coordinating your care is tremendously important to your well-being and the quality and safety of care you receive. You will have numerous health care encounters over time. The question is how will you track these health care experiences and how will you communicate them to all who should know your health history. We are not just passive participants in the process of coordinating our care. More and more, we will play an integral role in ensuring that coordination happens the way it needs to so we receive appropriate and safe medical care.

REFERENCES

1. Department of Health and Human Services. Summary of the HIPAA Privacy Rules. Available at: http://www.hhs.gov. Accessed October 30, 2013.

RESOURCES

- **HIPAA:** The regulations for protecting the privacy of your medical record data are described in HIPAA privacy (U. S. Department of Health and Human Services).

- **Medicare.gov:** This website is the official site for the U.S. government's Medicare program. It addresses issues of coverage, eligibility, benefits, and enrollments in Medicare.

TERMS

Coordinated Care: Coordinated care refers to the organization of patient care activities between two or more agencies including you, the patient. The goal is to achieve the most appropriate health care services.

Health Insurance Portability and Accountability Act (HIPAA): HIPAA regulations protect the privacy of the use, storage, maintenance, and transmission of health care patient data.

Medication Reconciliation: Medication reconciliation refers to the comparison of the patients list of current medications with those providers have, especially conducted at times of care transition e.g. with hospital admission, discharge and transfer orders. This process is used to ensure accuracy and patient safety.

Personal Health Record (PHR): Unlike either EHRs or EMRs, a PHR is a record with information about your health that you, or someone helping you, keeps. It can be as extensive as you want it to be.

Electronic Health Record (EHR): EHRs are centralized databases containing a comprehensive medical history and related information that can be shared across different health care system electronically.

Electronic Medical Record (EMR): EMRs are similar to EHRs and also play a significant role in coordinating care. Like EHRs, they are electronically collected, monitored, stored, and maintained. EMRs differ from EHRs in that they are generally less comprehensive, and are limited to the care provided to you by a single provider or provider group.

PART IV

- Your health care rights and responsibilities

- Using information resources and the internet wisely to know about your health and health care

CHAPTER 11

YOUR HEALTH CARE RIGHTS AND RESPONSIBILITIES

"There is the need to protect patient confidentiality and at the same time ensure the transmittal of medical information freely across health care sectors in the most timely fashion. How will we address the two simultaneously?"

The Author

WHAT YOU'LL FIND IN THIS CHAPTER:

- **GENERAL DESCRIPTION OF PATIENT RIGHTS IN HEALTH CARE**

- **THE PRIVILEDGED NATURE OF PATIENT-PROVIDER RELATIONSHIP**

- **PATIENT AND PROVIDER COMMUNICATIONS: ISSUES OF CONFIDENTIALITY, ANONYMITY, AND PRIVACY**

Why would you enter into an agreement with any institution without knowing that there are certain inalienable rights protecting you and your family? In many instances, these rights apply to your knowing exactly what services you will receive and what your rights are with respect to these services. The information presented here is to protect you from entering into an agreement where you won't like the results or sustaining risks that could hurt you. Health care providers are morally obligated to respect human existence and the individuality of all patients who are recipients of their care.

In health care, patients are protected in numerous ways through laws and regulations. These stipulate your rights, limit what providers can do, and the training necessary for medical practice. Today, most health care systems will have a statement of rights and obligations along with a list of your responsibilities along with a list of your responsibilities. Even insurance carriers (e.g. Blue Shield) post statements of member bill of rights with an attachment of patient responsibilities. Most of these publications are online on the institution's website. The foundation for patient rights in health care will be discussed further in this chapter.

GENERAL DESCRIPTION OF PATIENT RIGHTS IN HEALTH CARE

We live in an era of renewed protection of our rights for equitable health care. Health care reform policy now and always has been built on the premise that access to health care is not a privilege, but **A RIGHT**. There is ample evidence to prove a connection between lack of access to quality care and higher mortality and poor quality of life. Those unable to access care are most likely to die at an earlier age and suffer poor quality of life.

New health care reform requires insurance plans to cover preventive services and stops insurance companies from denying you coverage because you were previously ill or injured. The goal is to provide affordable health insurance for all U.S. citizens. There are other laws and stipulations that act in concert to ensure your individual rights when you are under the care of a health care provider. They will be discussed next.

THE PRIVILEGED NATURE OF PATIENT-PROVIDER RELATIONSHIP

Duty to the patient, including a breach of duty, underlies standards of practice for all health care professionals. When health care professionals enter into a relationship with a patient, a duty or obligation that is recognized as a legal relationship ensues. The provider has a duty to provide care.

Although providers can't deny a patient care, there are circumstances that will support providers who refuse to give care to some patients. These include physical risk. In this case, there is strong evidence to suggest more than minimal risk to providers if they care for a certain patient and any religious and/or moral issues that cause the provider to object to giving care.

Most institutions will support a provider's personal objections provided that these are stated well in advance and result in no harm or negative consequences for patients.

Perhaps the most noteworthy examples of professional-patient relationship privilege are embedded in the concepts of *informed choice* and *informed consent*. Informed choice ensures that you are given choices in the care you receive. Informed consent means that you are given all the information needed to make a decision.

In each and every health care situation, providers have a duty to offer you choices and participation in decisions that are important to your case. Health care decisions should be made on the basis of information about options. The decision that follows results in voluntary and informed decision- making. The parameters include both whether you want to receive health care and what method of procedure you choose. These choices are always reflective of the medical technology and resources available. For example, a provider cannot offer you an alternative surgical procedure if that procedure is contrary to good medical practice or is not available due to lack of well trained medical staff. Providers are, however, obligated to describe the alternatives that are available, if not with them, then in other treatment centers. Informed choice requires providers to clearly communicate about the best treatment but also about other less-favored approaches.

The principle of informed consent is closely related to informed choice. Informed consent occurs after you have obtained full information about the nature of medical procedures or treatment that is recommended to you by your provider. Not only must you be told the nature of the treatment or procedure, you must understand any risks or benefits associated with the treatment. Your consent must not be obtained through misrepresentation of information or deceit. You can't be coerced to give consent.

Sometimes, providers perform this task ineffectively and options are not fully and adequately discussed. Providers may appear as if they are pressuring you one way or another. Their encounters with you or your family may suggest that if you fail to follow their advice, there may be negative repercussions. This type of response from a provider is unacceptable and unethical. A patient's fear of abandonment or retaliation, real or imagined, can influence whether he or she will exercise his or her autonomous decision-making. Fears could include concerns that the treatment you receive will be withdrawn, will be of lesser quality, or that you will suffer unnecessary pain or discomfort. If providers don't discuss with you the choices available, you can't effectively participate in decision-making.

Despite the subtle, and sometimes not so subtle, interplay between providers' preference and patients' choices, one thing must be clear: *You, the patient, are the primary decision-maker*. It is generally maintained that you are a critical participant and should retain significant control over health care decisions that affect your welfare.

PATIENT RIGHTS TO CONFIDENTIALITY, ANONYMITY, AND PRIVACY

A number of important concepts surround patient rights to confidentiality. Over the years, much attention has focused on the scope of patient rights as they apply to *confidentiality* and *privacy of information*. The ethical codes of professional organizations aim to safeguard your right to protect information you offer in encounters with health care providers.

RIGHT TO CONFIDENTIALITY

Paticnt confidcntially has its basis in vcry carly law. In our country, the right to confidentiality and privacy is supported by the Fourth Amendment to the U.S. Constitution: *"The right of the people to be secure in their persons, houses, papers, and effects, against unreasonable searches and seizures"*. Under law, this right may not be violated.

Health providers have a duty to keep in confidence whatever you tell them or whatever they might learn about you while caring for you. It is undcrstood that thc naturc of thc paticnt-providcr rclationship will reveal private information about you. Some of this information you may not have been aware of its existence. This is due to the trust you place on this helping relationship and the intensive exploration of a wide variety of issues that influence your health and which information must be retrieved to treat you properly. When you seek medical intervention, you are asked to reveal very intimate details about yourself and your family. These may be things that no one else knows. Examples of this would be: your basic fears and concerns, use of illicit drugs, your sexual practices, and your attitude about whether life is worth living. In fact, effective patient-provider relationships rely on your willingness and ability to talk frankly and openly about these situations. The information may be denunciatory or incriminating.

Confidentiality has the sole purpose of protecting you from unauthorized disclosures. It is the patient's basic right to have his/her privacy respected. This privacy can't be breached. Only patients have the right to release information in their medical record. That is why you are frequently asked to sign for release of medical information to your insurance company or to another health care provider. The American Medical Association clearly states that any breach in confidentiality no matter how minor, can be construed as a grounds for mistrust and potential litigation and disciplinary action.[1]

The guarantee of confidentiality also applies to your written medical records. That is, your provider has the obligation and duty to maintain your records in a manner in which there is no reasonable chance of their getting lost, stolen, or falling into the hands of unauthorized persons. With the advent of electronic health records and e-mails between provider and patient, interpretations and guidelines are not so straightforward, but are becoming more explicit out of the need to transfer important data in a timely manner.

Let's consider some typical examples where your right to confidentiality would not be protected.

CONSIDER THE FOLLOWING:

Your doctor gives another doctor your name because he/she thinks you need a consultation. This is before you give the referring doctor your permission. Not only that, your doctor reveals to the other doctor that you have a diagnosis of cervical cancer. You have not been told about your diagnosis, and therefore, your rights have been violated. Your doctor divulged information without your permission and breached the rules of confidentiality. Professional ethics would support the sanctioning of any health care provider who violated your rights to confidentiality.

There are some exceptions. Many states have granted statutes that guarantee privileged communication but have been challenged by arguments against privileged communication. A case in point for example might center around whether this information is critical in protecting the health and welfare of others. It is essential to reveal certain health information that would otherwise be held confidential because reporting it is essential to protect society. A most notable example where the rights to confidentiality were challenged was in a landmark case in California (Tarasoff v. Regents of the University of California, 1974). This case set an important precedent in the U.S. and many other parts of the world. The critical incident involved a psychotherapist knowing that a patient had homicidal thoughts toward a specific person but did not warn the person who was in danger. The situation resulted in the stabbing to death of the targeted person. This landmark case established that despite otherwise preservation of patient-provider communications, it was a therapist's duty to warn *endangered parties.*

RIGHT TO ANONYMITY AND PRIVACY

Anonymity refers to your right to have your identity protected from its being known to others. Consider the following three examples:

- A pharmacist assistant speaks loudly to a person in the presence of several other people standing in line to pick up your medications: "Mr. Smith, your antidepressant is ready for pick up." This specific information is about medications also includes your diagnosis. This would be a violation of your rights even if no one in line recognizes what an antidepressant is, or even knows you by name.
- Another example of breach of confidentiality is if providers were discussing the details of a patient's condition, revealing a first or last name while riding in the office building elevator. If you witness such events you will notice that onlookers like yourself will turn their heads and look down or look away. People are aware

that this data is privileged and that they are not really supposed to know this information.

- A patient in an outpatient clinic is awaiting diagnostic-testing procedures. The receptionist broadcasts the name of the patient to the room of six to seven other patients and family members. Having not obtained all the information initially, she requests the patient to call back to her (behind the desk) the reason for the diagnostic test, where the patient lives, and home and work phone numbers. This can be embarrassing to patients and is a violation of their confidentiality.

Can we say that it is ok to reveal this information publicly? Every patient, including you, who experiences a violation has the opportunity to file a health information privacy complaint with the Office for Civil Rights (OCR). Given the rights of patients for anonymity and privacy, this information *is* confidential and should not be discussed openly. These infractions are serious ethical errors. Is it worth suing the provider, assistant, and/or health care facility? Not really. The breach of health privacy is governed by federal law the Health Insurance Portability and Accountability Act (HIPAA). There is no civil lawsuit provision with this federal law. However, these violations are investigated by the OCR, Department of Health and Human Services. This violation could be reported to the violator's state board of professional practice. However, in the case described, the violation was committed by a nonprofessional staff member.

There are numerous documents that you will sign in the process of receiving medical care. Read them carefully. You will see that some of these documents testify to the fact that your rights as a patient are being protected and your concurrent responsibilities are recognized. These documents are given to you when you become a new patient and when you are consenting to a procedure, surgical intervention, or hospitalization. These documents attest to your rights for complete, current information concerning your diagnosis, treatment, and prognosis in terms that you can be reasonably expected to understand. Except in emergencies when you lack decision-making capacity and the need for treatment is urgent, you are entitled to the opportunity to discuss and request information related to the specific procedures and/or treatments, the risks involved, the possible length of recuperation, and the medically reasonable alternatives and their accompanying risks and benefits.

Perhaps the most dramatic example of the shift to provide patients with information is seen in the following example. Not more than two decades ago it was unthinkable for patients to exercise their rights to the extent of requesting copies of everything in their medical record, including notes, lab-test results, doctors' orders, and so forth. Today, it is a patient right. This request occurs, albeit infrequently, and while the entire chart is not usually provided, excerpts of the contents of the record are summarized for you. This request is not only for the purpose of completing referrals, it is in response to a direct request of patients to have access records. In your files you should find copies of signed consent forms to indicate that you were properly informed and have consented to treatment.

In summary, a lack of effective communication between you and your providers is often at the root of violations of your rights as a patient if they occur. Your providers have an obligation to care and protect you from harm. If you do not know what your treatment options are, are not aware of the consequences of a chosen treatment, or feel that the choice provided is not a "real choice," your rights as a patient may be in jeopardy.

REFERENCES

1. American Medical Association (AMA). Patient Confidentiality. Division of Health Law. May 07, 1007. Available at: http://www.ama-assn.org/ama/pub/category/4610.html. Accessed November 1, 2013.

RESOURCES

- Patient's Bill of Rights, American Hospital Association (October 21, 1992). In a subsequent document the American Hospital Association (AHA) drafted a newer document referred to as: The Patient Care Partnership. Available at: http://www.aha.org/aha/content/2003/pdf/pcp_english_030730.pdf. Accessed October 14, 2008.

TERMS

Advance Directives: Advance Directives specify your instructions to others about how you want to handle your health care. They also allow you to name a person to make health care decisions on your behalf if you are not able to do so. When you are admitted to a hospital you generally will be asked if you have an advance directive.

Informed Choice: Patients who have the capacity to make decisions about their health care have the right to do so.

Informed Consent: Informed consent is the consent patients give to have treatments, procedures, or tests performed. In a few cases it may be obtained orally but most likely in writing.

Rights to Anonymity and Privacy: Anonymity refers to the right to protection of identity whereas privacy refers to patients' rights to limit what others know about them.

Right to Confidentiality: Patients have the right to have personal information about them held in confidence and not disclosed unless permission is given. Providers have an ethical and legal responsibility to protect the confidentiality of patient information.

Self-Determination: Self-determination or freedom of choice refers to the patient's right to accept or refuse medical treatment.

CHAPTER 12

USING INFORMATION RESOURCES AND THE INTERNET WISELY TO KNOW ABOUT YOUR HEALTH AND HEALTH CARE

"More than half of Americans access health information on the internet...the problem is in knowing the quality of this information."

The Author

WHAT YOU'LL FIND IN THIS CHAPTER:

- **WARNING SIGNS ABOUT INFORMATION ON THE WEB**

- **A DESCRIPTION OF THE VARIETY OF INFORMATION AVAILABLE**

- **HOW TO EVALUATE THE QUALITY OF WEB INFORMATION**

- **HOW TO INTERACT WITH YOUR PROVIDER ABOUT INFORMATION ON THE WEB**

There is a wealth of information available to you on the World Wide Web. In most cases, this information will help you participate actively in your health care. The quality of this information varies and it is best that you learn what is available and how to evaluate the quality of information. This chapter will describe the range of information on the web, teach you the principles of evaluating information on the web, provide you a list of quality web sites and trustworthy sources, and how to interact with your provider after obtaining this kind of information.

WARNING SIGNS ABOUT USING WEB SITES

While some of us are still uncomfortable with using the internet, the fact is we are using it more often. The most frequent use is to obtain information dealing with health and health care.

Your access to health information on the internet has the potential of increasing your knowledge of what concerns you, and therefore better prepares you to act as an active collaborator in your primary care. However, there are limitations to the quality of information available on many sites and you are going to need to know how to be wise consumers of this information.

YOU MUST REMEMBER THAT THE INFORMATION YOU ACCESS ON THE WEB DOES NOT TAKE THE PLACE OF THE ADVICE YOU GET FROM A PRIMARY HEALTH CARE PROVIDER!
ALSO
ANY ADVICE GIVEN TO YOU IN THE ABSENSE OF THIS PROVIDER REALLY KNOWING YOUR CASE AND CONDUCTING A FULL MEDICAL ASSESSMENT IS INADEQUATE!

Let's discuss the first warning. There are some of us who enjoy searching the web for just about anything we want to know. There is a certain personal empowerment in figuring something out on our own. Much of this type of learning occurs in isolation. This process raises problems. For example, you may go online and read about how dangerous some medications are (e.g. antidepressants, statins, or drugs to treat osteoporosis, like Actonel).

You might decide that you shouldn't take them and you cut back on the dose. This is your attempt to make them "safer" or more tolerable. The problem is you (and your provider) are no longer treating your condition the way it should be treated. Another example would include deciding that the symptoms you have do not match what is described online. You decide that you don't have depression; rather, you are suffering from chronic fatigue syndrome. If you fail to tell your provider how you think about your symptoms and what you are doing, you are creating even more problems.

One of the original concerns that the American Medical Association (AMA) had about the internet was the consequence of the public believing that what they read was trustworthy and something that could be applied to them. The organization cautioned that there was a great variation in the information provided and that without the details reviewed under the care of the physician, this information was not meant to be used freely and carelessly.

Just as important is if the provider receives an email from the patient, and then analyzes the case and answers the patient. This activity is unethical because it offers diagnostic data without the provider ever seeing the patient or reviewing medical records needed in making a thorough assessment. It should be noted that this situation is different from a patient and provider discussing care issues over emails when the health and treatment of the patient is an ongoing process with the identified provider.

Using internet information to learn about your health and medical care has increased significantly. The American Medical Association (AMA) cautioned patients not to overuse this information because it was believed the relationship with physicians would change and patients would be exposed to inaccurate details about their conditions.

The assumption was that this information would misguide patients and cause them to rely less on professional judgments of licensed health care providers. These assumptions have not been proven to be true in every case; instead, providers have learned to appreciate the fact that exposure to internet information has caused patients to be more inquisitive and ready for active participation in health care decisions.

A DESCRIPTION OF THE VARIETY OF INFORMATION AVAILABLE

There are several avenues for gaining health information and support through the use of the internet. These include: 1) email communications, (2) community information (e.g. the use of bulletin boards, chat rooms, and electronic counseling and support groups), and (3) health information content found in professional journal articles and technical reports. Patients who once relied heavily on friends, family, newspapers, magazines, and on health providers, to a lesser extent, can now turn to the internet for a wide range of health and medical care knowledge. The health care delivery system itself has spurned this change. The inability to access information from a real provider in a timely manner has made the internet attractive.

The majority of us who are using the internet for health information are searching online for information about a specific disease or medical problem. This would be about common chronic illnesses (e.g. Cancer, heart disease, stroke, arthritis, and diabetes), as well as injuries (e.g. burns, abrasions, and broken limbs), and infections (e.g. urinary and pulmonary infections).

In addition to this disease-specific interest, early on there was an increase in what web information could be found about a variety of health related topics (e.g. diet/nutrition, fitness, health insurance, and alternative therapies). There was also interest in information about hospitals, medical providers, and experimental treatments. These topics have been expanded to include information about specific medications, over-the-counter drugs and illness prevention. Now the internet offers not only information about patient care, but the opportunity for you to gain long term support in adjusting to and managing your care. Virtual communities in the form of blogs, chat rooms, discussion groups, and email exchanges exist. The magnitude of opportunities is overwhelming. But the chance of picking up bad advice or inaccurate information is also compounded. It is important for you to beware of both the advantages and drawbacks that might occur.

Before we leave this topic it is important to describe the growing interest in patient-led websites that may be very useful. The opportunity to communicate with others in the same situation makes an important contribution. When confronting an acute or chronic condition, we frequently have the need to talk to other people who really understand what it is like. Participation in a virtual community might be our only option to satisfy these important needs. Let's take the example of a woman who is coping with the demands of treatment for breast cancer. Topics on virtual communities (e.g. through blogs or chat rooms can include how to manage the stress and physical discomfort, talk to their family about their condition, maintain intimacy with their mates, and deal with the stigma and fear generated in others). Here is the partial discussion of a breast cancer patient who has been in remission for over six years and is using a patient-led support network on the web:

"When I talk to other people about my cancer they always say '..... but look how far you have come....you are five years out without any symptoms...you should be feeling good'. They don't understand that we are always waiting for the 'next shoe to drop'." The patient knows that while others do not understand her ongoing fears...the patients on this supportive website are more likely to. With this support she feels more validated and less 'crazy'. These kinds of discussions through the internet are clearly valuable for many reasons. They offer support but also information from others who have been through similar circumstances. There is a real possibility that these patients could learn from others what their providers told them, but they didn't understand.

Gwen van Servellen RN PhD

How To Evaluate The Quality Of Web Information

Not all patients have access to the internet and an even smaller number have the ability to sort through this information and determine what is usable and what is not. It is important that we all get access and are guided in how to use the information on line. Patients need to know how to protect themselves from misinformation. Your providers may not always have the time to counsel you about health and medical information on the internet so it is imperative that you learn as much as you can. Information on the internet is constantly changing and much of it is being updated frequently; thus, to become a real consumer it is best to keep going back to what you read and evaluate if any changes or additions that have been made.

The growth in the use of the internet has raised additional concerns. Not all of us have access to learning from the web and not all of us have the skills and motivation for learning how best to sort through good and not so good internet advice. The term used to designate the unequal preparation in our communities is: *digital divide*. This refers to the fact that some of us are very prepared to search and judge online information and others of us are not; hence, the internet further builds a wedge between those of us who receive good medical information and those of who do not. The problem of sorting through information on the internet also raises the point that not all of this information is directed for lay person use. Much of it is directed at professional health care providers. Some data requires interpretation by persons with certain academic credentials, especially when the reports use scientific evidence and statistics. Additionally, much of the information is provided in English only, presenting further problems to patients whose primary language is not English. Also, a significant problem rests in the patient's misinterpretation of information provided.

Some websites are maintained by interest groups and may market products (e.g. pharmaceutical companies and weight loss programs).

However, there are many well-respected sites (e.g. the American Cancer Society and the American Heart Association) that can be trusted.

The following are general guidelines that might help you. The first thing you must know is what questions are you interested in being answered (e.g. do I have symptoms of arthritis?). Secondly, where do you want to start? Do you want to do a narrow search of existing websites or do you want to do a broad search of all existing information on the internet? If you are familiar with search engines, this is another place to start. Enter your topic (e.g. symptoms of arthritis) and look at the information sites found. There will be numerous. Still another approach is to go into a trusted and well-respected website that deals specifically with conditions that you are interested in. In the case of arthritis, this would be the National Institute of Arthritis and Musculoskeletal and Skin Diseases.

Let's use another specific example. Let's say you want to know whether green tea helps in preventing cancers. Herbal preparations, with either green or black tea, have been studied for their properties to protect the public from cancer and also as complementary treatments when someone is diagnosed with cancer. Some patients may want to know if drinking green tea might slow the progression of cancer while they are still undergoing conventional cancer treatment. What type of search of the web would you conduct? If you say a broad search of the literature you may not be on the right track. This approach will yield a lot of extraneous information and much of it might be irrelevant or conflicted. It will be time consuming and you may not trust your ability to weed through the accuracy of the information before you.

Because of the potential of ending up with the wrong information or no clear information or direction, the best route is to go directly to the National Institutes for information. This would be the National Cancer Institute. A second option would be to go to the American Cancer Society. If you didn't take this advice and decided to perform a broad search you would be confronted with thousands of resources. Try it and see what happens. So you did try it and you learned that indeed there are thousands of resources.

Some of these extraneous resources may be of interest to you or may also be helpful in answering your questions. But here is why the American Cancer Society (ACS) and National Cancer Institute (NCI) will be preferable. These sites will have the latest information on your topic or they will be able to refer you to sources that would be helpful. You will have the option of searching many topics, including the latest treatments for specific cancers, how to get quality medical care, and stories of hope and inspiration written by cancer survivors. It is recommended that you first go to the ACS and NCI sites.

How To Interact With Your Provider About Information On The Web

In general, you are likely to seek on-line information before seeing your provider, not to challenge your provider's wisdom or knowledge, but to improve your own. After your visit with your provider you might go back to the information you gained on the internet. This could give you reassurance if what your provider said is exactly what was written online. Or, if the information is different, then you might have more questions to ask your provider during your next office visit.

Some providers, if they have an email address, receive unsolicited emails from the public looking for advice, but these individuals do not have a pre-existing relationship with the provider. As previously described, in this instance the provider is placed in a compromising situation. By law, they can't offer a diagnosis or recommendation for treatment. It is unethical and against the law to diagnose and treat people over the internet in the absence of a pre-existing patient-provider relationship.

There are recent approaches that are ethical and are used in treating and maintaining connections with patients. One approach is "telemedicine". Telemedicine is the process of gaining medical information and sharing it more widely via electronic means. It includes a variety of services including video conferencing, smart phone use, and patient communications through the use of distant health buddy networks to keep providers informed about their symptoms.

In this case, patients who do not have easy access to health services due to their residential location (e.g. rural areas) or for reasons of disability (e.g. they are home-bound), will benefit greatly by telemedicine programs. Still, medical providers will have to meet certain safety criteria to ensure that care is high quality and that the patient is fully informed.

Despite the fact that you are probably not looking to challenge your provider's thinking and decision-making, this does not mean that all providers will welcome your new-found knowledge gleamed from the internet. First, they may not know the web source you are quoting, the information you present, and may not understand why you are presenting the data. Be prepared and not surprised. Yes, there may be some providers who just want you to accept their opinion and not bother them with other points of view. But, more likely than not, and depending upon the way you present it, most providers would welcome your eagerness to become involved. They would show you that they are open to this information especially if another one of their patients is likely to ask for a discussion using the same information.

There is still another potential provider response. Some providers could recommend selected websites to you. In this case, the provider is probably very familiar with the site and has read the material before recommending it to others. In this case providers will have pre-judged the likelihood that you would easily understand it and that it is relevant to your concerns. Providers may even take the time to explain why they chose the site for you and how to evaluate other internet sites covering the same material.

When you present internet information to your providers you should expect them to respond with openness and gratitude. They should show interest in the information as well as the source of the information, receive your request to discuss the information as a positive sign that you want to be an active participant, and direct you to other sites which have high quality information.

In summary, a growing number of patients bring internet based health care information to their providers. These conversations are likely to increase as you familiarize yourself with the data that is available on the internet. The use of the internet remains a barrier for those who have no access or for other reasons (age, health, literacy, linguistic, and socioeconomic status) lack the ability to search and screen for quality information. This is an important role for family health care providers. It is hoped that this chapter will encourage you to try the internet, but also involve your family members in helping you. Be sure to use those trusted and well-respected websites available to you and your family.

REFERENCES

1. Lopez L, Green AR. et al. Bridging the digital divide in health care: the role of health information technology in addressing racial and ethnic disparities. Joint Commission *J Qual Patient Saf.* 37(10): 437-445.

RESOURCES

Figure 1. Recommended Internet Sites for Evaluating Health Care Information

INTERNET RESOURCES	HELP PROVIDED
THE HEALTH INFORMATION QUALITY ASSESSMENT TOOL (hitiweb.mitretek.org/lg)	This service provides a tool for evaluating internet sites. The tool helps you to determine their credibility.

HEALTH INSIGHT: TAKING CHARGE OF HEALTH INFORMATION (Harvard School of Public Health)	This guide seeks to help consumers evaluate health and scientific information and consider how the information can be used to improve their lives
HEALTH ON THE WEB: FINDING RELIABLE INFORMATION (American Academy of Family Physicians)	This site outlines several important criteria to judge information on the web.
HOW TO EVALUATE HEALTH INFORMATION ON THE INTERNET (NIH: National Center for Complementary and Alternative Medicine)	This website presents and discusses scientific evidence about the use of complementary health approaches.
USER'S GUIDE TO FINDING AND EVALUATING HEALTH INFORMATION ON THE WEB (NIH: U.S. National Library of Medicine)	This website is for consumers looking for health information. It helps you to find and evaluate information on the web.

TEN THINGS TO KNOW ABOUT EVALUATING MEDICAL RESOURCES ON THE WEB (NIH: National Center For Complementary and Alternative Medicine)	This is a short guide containing important questions to consider when looking for health information online and focuses on Complementary and Alternative Medicine.
TEN TIPS FOR EVALUATING IMMUNIZATION INFORMATION ON THE INTERNET (Centers for Disease Control and Prevention)	This is a short guide containing important questions to consider when looking for information online about immunizations.
UNDERSTANDING RISK: WHAT DO THOSE HEADLINES REALLY MEAN? (NIH: National Institutes of Health, National Institute on Aging)	This website provides a fact sheet that will help you evaluate news reports you read in the newspaper or see on television about medical studies and the interpretation of these studies' findings.
GATEWAY SITE: HEALTHFINDER (www.healthfinder.gov/)	Source for reliable health information from the Federal government. It offers quick guides to healthy living, personalized health advice based upon your age and gender.

AMERICAN MEDICAL ASSOCIATION (Medem.com)	Provides access to consumer related information published by the National Institutes of Health. NIH search engine is also available on this site.
NATIONAL INSTITUTES BY DISEASE AND CONDITION (NATIONAL CANCER INSTITUTE, NATIONAL INSTITUTE ON AGING, NATIONAL INSTITUTE OF ARTHRITIS AND MUSCULOSKELETAL AND SKIN DISEASES)	These sites provide a wide array of medical information and offer the same news and information available at online health channels. They provide access to disease and illness prevention and treatment specific information, including recent research and clinical trials.

TERMS

Digital Divide: This term is used to designate the unequal preparation in our communities to access, understand and use information on the internet. Some of us are very prepared to search and judge online information and others of us are not; hence, the internet further builds a wedge between those of us who receive good medical information and those of who do not.

Telemedicine: Telemedicine is an approach to stay in continuous communication with patients about their care. It is the process of gaining medical information and sharing it more widely via electronic means. Telemedicine includes a variety of services including video conferencing, smart phone use, and patient communications through the use of distant health buddy networks to keep providers informed about their symptoms.

Virtual Community: The internet offers a number of opportunities to create online communities in the form of blogs, chat rooms, discussion groups, and email exchanges. These communities are not geographical entities but nonetheless exist in cyberspace to offer patients support and information.

ABOUT THE AUTHOR

Gwen van Servellen, RN, PhD is a nationally and internationally recognized educator, consultant, and author. She is a UCLA Professor Emeritus who has spent over 35 years evaluating patient care in both inpatient and outpatient settings. Dr. van Servellen has consulted with hospitals, clinics and outpatient centers, and universities in the United States and around the world.

As an author she has published over 100 professional articles and conference proceedings and 7 books on the topics of individualized care, healthcare processes and cost effectiveness, quality care, and effective communications between patients and health professionals.

Prior to this book, she wrote textbooks for health care professionals on the topic of health care communications. Dr. van Servellen's motivation is to prepare professionals and consumers simultaneously in hopes that this synergy will help them work together to achieve quality health care within and outside the borders of the hospital.

Having been an observer and recipient of both "good" and "bad" care she is particularly interested in helping you overcome any challenges you might face in getting high levels of quality healthcare.

To learn more about Gwen van Servellen and resources for getting the most from your healthcare visit: www.HealthCareBooks.net

Special offer for readers of this book:

Get these two free reports by visiting

www.HealthCareBooks.net/bonus

Common Medical Errors That Can Harm or Kill You

Why Hospital Infections Happen and How to Avoid Getting One

68067907R10113

Made in the USA
San Bernardino, CA
30 January 2018